Fractures of the Foot and Ankle

Nirmal C. Tejwani
Editor

Fractures of the Foot and Ankle

A Clinical Casebook

Springer

Editor
Nirmal C. Tejwani
Department of Orthopedic Surgery
NYU Langone Medical Center
New York, NY
USA

ISBN 978-3-319-60455-8 ISBN 978-3-319-60456-5 (eBook)
DOI 10.1007/978-3-319-60456-5

Library of Congress Control Number: 2017951867

Printed on acid-free paper

This Springer imprint is published by Springer Nature
The registered company is Springer International Publishing AG
The registered company address is: Gewerbestrasse 11, 6330 Cham, Switzerland

This book is dedicated to my wife Mona and my daughters Ruchi and Rhea, as it would not have been possible without their support and encouragement.

Preface

Injuries to the foot and ankle are common and a wide variety of implants and techniques are available for their surgical treatment. This is based on fracture type and location, soft tissue status, implant availability as well as surgeon experience. With the spectrum of injuries ranging from intra-articular fractures to complex combinations of injuries, the treatment methods vary widely. Use of internal or external fixation is described using actual cases as treated by the authors.

The purpose of this book is to give the readers case examples of different foot and ankle fractures from the ankle to the metatarsals and their treatment options. This book is entirely case based and uses clinical case scenarios and attempts to put you in the surgeon's shoes. Each case illustrates different options for treatment with the author's thinking process; follow-up and outcomes of options used in the treatment are also reported. The goal is not to substitute knowledge learning from textbooks or journals but to provide clinical examples elucidating the translation of theory to practice.

The reader must be aware that not all of these treatment options may be applicable to all situations, but will hopefully make you aware of what is possible.

The creation of this book would have been impossible without the conceptual insight of Kristopher Spring (Editor, Clinical Medicine) and the logistical support of Kumar Athiappan (Development Editor), both at Springer. Much gratitude is owed to them for their professionalism and engagement that resulted in the timely execution of the book project.

New York, USA — Nirmal C. Tejwani

Contents

Contributors

Jaimo Ahn, MD, PhD, FACS Department of Orthopaedic Surgery, University of Pennsylvania, Philadelphia, PA, USA

Michael T. Archdeacon, MD, MSE Department of Orthopaedic Surgery, University of Cincinnati Academic Health Center, Cincinnati, OH, USA

Mark Ayoub, MD Department of Orthopaedic Surgery, Rutgers-Robert Wood Johnson University Hospital, New Brunswick, NJ, USA

Chad Beck, MD Medical College of Wisconsin, 9200 W. Wisconsin Ave, Milwaukee, WI, USA

Clayton C. Bettin, MD Department of Orthopaedic Surgery, University of Tennessee—Campbell Clinic, Memphis, TN, USA

Amrut Borade, MBBS, MS Department of Orthopaedics, Geisinger Health System, Danville, PA, USA

Alexander M. Crespo, MD Orthopedic Surgery, NYU Hospital for Joint Diseases, New York, NY, USA

Natalie R. Danna, MD Department of Orthopedics, NYU Langone Medical Center, New York, NY, USA

Roy I. Davidovitch, MD Orthopedic Surgery, NYU Hospital for Joint Diseases, New York, NY, USA

J. Dheenadhayalan, MS (Ortho) Department of Orthopaedics, Ganga Hospital, Coimbatore, India

Tonya L. Dixon, MD, MPH Department of Orthopaedic Surgery, Division of Foot and Ankle Surgery, Massachusetts General Hospital, Waltham, MA, USA

Mark Gage, MD Department of Orthopaedics, University of Maryland School of Medicine, R. Adams Cowley Shock Trauma Center, Baltimore, MD, USA

Abhishek Ganta, MD Department of Orthopaedic Surgery, Hospital for Joint Diseases, New York University School of Medicine, New York, NY, USA

Department of Orthopaedic Surgery, NYU Hospital for Joint Diseases, NYU Langone Medical Center, New York, NY, USA

Daniel J. Gittings, MD Department of Orthopaedic Surgery, University of Pennsylvania, Philadelphia, PA, USA

Nikhil A. Gokhale, MS (Orth.), MRCS (Ed.) Registrar in Orthopaedics, Trauma and Orthopaedics, Kings Mill Hospital, Sherwood Forest Hospitals, NHS Foundation Trust, Sutton in Ashfield, Nottinghamshire, UK

Mitch Harris, MD Orthopaedic Surgery, Brigham and Women's Hospital, Boston, MA, USA

Marilyn Heng, MD, MPH, FRCSC Orthopaedic Surgery, Massachusetts General Hospital, Harvard Orthopaedic Trauma Initiative, Boston, MA, USA

Daniel Scott Horwitz, MD Department of Orthopaedics, Geisinger Health System, Danville, PA, USA

Harish Kempegowda, MBBS, MS Department of Orthopaedics, Geisinger Health System, Danville, PA, USA

Sanjit R. Konda, MD Jamaica Hospital Medical Center, Queens, NY, USA

Department of Orthopaedic Surgery, NYU Langone Medical Center, NYU Hospital for Joint Diseases, New York, NY, USA

Philipp Leucht, MD Department of Orthopaedic Surgery, Hospital for Joint Diseases, New York University School of Medicine, New York, NY, USA

Frank A. Liporace, MD Department of Orthopaedic Surgery, Jersey City Medical Center—RWJBarnabas Health, Jersey City, NJ, USA

Matthew S. MacDougall, MS Department of Biochemistry and Molecular Genetics, University of Illinois, Chicago, IL, USA

Toni M. McLaurin, MD Department of Orthopaedic Surgery, Chief of Orthopaedic Service Bellevue Hospital Center, NYU Langone Medical Center, New York, NY, USA

William Min, MD, MS, MBA The Hughston Clinic at Gwinnett Medical Center, Lawrenceville, GA, USA

Kenneth J. Mroczek, MD Department of Orthopedic Surgery, New York University Langone Hospital for Joint Diseases, New York, NY, USA

Florian Nickisch, MD Department of Orthopaedic Surgery, University of Utah School of Medicine, Salt Lake City, UT, USA

Kathryn O'Connor, MD, MSPT Department of Orthopaedics, University of Pennsylvania, Philadelphia, PA, USA

Selene G. Parekh, MD, MBA Department of Orthopaedic Surgery, Duke University Medical Center, Durham, NC, USA

Edward A. Perez, MD Department of Orthopaedic Surgery, University of Tennessee—Campbell Clinic, Memphis, TN, USA

David Polonet, MD Department of Orthopaedic Surgery, Jersey Shore University Medical Center, Wall, NJ, USA

Saqib Rehman, MD Department of Orthopaedic Surgery, Temple University, Philadelphia, PA, USA

Megan Reilly, MD Department of Orthopaedic Surgery, Temple University, Philadelphia, PA, USA

Daniela Sanchez, MD Department of Orthopaedics, Geisinger Health System, Danville, PA, USA

Neil Sardesai, MD Department of Orthopaedics, University of Maryland School of Medicine, R. Adams Cowley Shock Trauma Center, Baltimore, MD, USA

Marcus Sciadini, MD Department of Orthopaedics, University of Maryland School of Medicine, R. Adams Cowley Shock Trauma Center, Baltimore, MD, USA

Daniel Segina, MD Department of Orthopaedic Surgery, Holmes Regional Medical Center, Melbourne, FL, USA

Rajiv Shah, MS (Ortho) Department of Foot and Ankle Orthopaedics, Sunshine Global Hospitals, Vadodara, India

Sunil M. Shahane, MS (Orth.), MCh (Orth.) Senior Orthopaedic Consultant, Orthopaedic and Trauma Surgery, Nanavati Super Speciality Hospital, Mumbai, Maharashtra, India

Brendan R. Southam, MD Department of Orthopaedic Surgery, University of Cincinnati Academic Health Center, Cincinnati, OH, USA

Nicole M. Stevens, MD Department of Orthopaedic Surgery, NYU Hospital for Joint Diseases, New York, NY, USA

Nirmal C. Tejwani, MD Department of Orthopedics, NYU Langone Medical Center, New York, NY, USA

Michael J. Weaver, MD Orthopaedic Surgery, Brigham and Women's Hospital, Boston, MA, USA

Ryan Wilson, PA-C, MPAS Department of Orthopaedics, Holmes Regional Medical Center, Melbourne, FL, USA

Philip Wolinsky, MD UC Davis Medical Center, Sacramento, CA, USA

Richard S. Yoon, MD Department of Orthopaedic Surgery, Jersey City Medical Center—RWJBarnabas Health, Jersey City, NJ, USA

Chapter 1
Unimalleolar Ankle Fracture: Lateral Malleolus Only/ Supination External Rotation (SER) 4

Toni M. McLaurin and Abhishek Ganta

Clinical History

A 64-year-old female with well-controlled type II diabetes and a history of prior transient ischemic attacks (TIAs) sustained an injury to her right ankle when she slipped and fell on ice. She noted immediate right ankle pain and deformity, was unable to bear weight after her fall, and presented to the emergency room. The patient had diffuse swelling and ecchymosis throughout her ankle and tenderness to palpation over the lateral malleolus. There was no tenderness medially. She was neurovascularly intact.

T.M. McLaurin, M.D. (✉)
Department of Orthopaedic Surgery, Chief of Orthopaedic Service
Bellevue Hospital Center, NYU Langone Medical Center,
550 First Avenue, BHC CD4-98, New York, NY 10016, USA
e-mail: toni.mclaurin@nyumc.org

A. Ganta, M.D.
Department of Orthopaedic Surgery, NYU Hospital
for Joint Diseases, NYU Langone Medical Center,
301 E. 17th Street, New York, NY 10003, USA

N.C. Tejwani (ed.), *Fractures of the Foot and Ankle*,
DOI 10.1007/978-3-319-60456-5_1,

Injury Radiographs

Anteroposterior (AP), lateral, and mortise views of the ankle demonstrate a long oblique lateral malleolus fracture at the level of the syndesmosis (Fig. 1.1). There is minimal comminution at the fracture site and the fracture extends in an anteroinferior to posterosuperior direction from the level of the plafond. The lateral view of the ankle demonstrates a comminuted posterior malleolus fracture that involves less than 10% of the articular surface. The mortise view shows an incongruent tibiotalar joint with lateral subluxation of the talus within the mortise. Given the direction and pattern of the fibula fracture, this patient was diagnosed with a Lauge-Hansen supination external rotation IV ankle fracture (SER IV).

There are several radiographic criteria used to assess tibiotalar and syndesmotic stability that must be evaluated on initial injury radiographs. These parameters include fibular shortening, widening of the medial joint space, talar tilt, and malrotation of the fibula. Adequately assessing the congruency of the tibiotalar articular is paramount as 1 mm of tibiotalar displacement can lead to a 40% increase in joint contact pressures [1]. While bimalleolar fractures are inherently unstable, an isolated fibula fracture is only considered unstable if there is an accompanying medial-sided deltoid ligament injury.

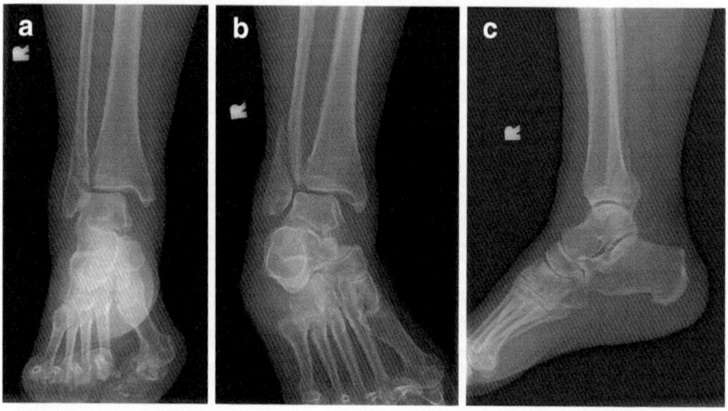

Figure 1.1 Anteroposterior (**a**), mortise (**b**), and lateral (**c**) radiographs showing an oblique lateral malleolus fracture with an intact medial malleolus and widening of the medial clear space on the AP and mortise views

Medial clear space widening of greater than or equal to 5 mm on radiographs taken in dorsiflexion with an external rotation stress is most predictive of deep deltoid ligament incompetence after a distal fibular fracture [2]. A stress external rotation radiograph done either manually or with gravity is obtained to determine if there is talar shift and often shows a high rate of positive stress on isolated fibular fractures with an intact mortise [3]. It is important to note that medial tenderness, ecchymosis, and swelling are *not* predictive of deltoid incompetence. Studies have shown that the use of gravity stress radiographs is equivalent to manual stress to determine medial-sided ligamentous injury [4]. However, the author's preference is to perform a manual stress examination.

Treatment Considerations and Timing of Surgery

Given the closed nature of this injury, after closed reduction and splinting, the decision was made to send the patient home and surgery was scheduled for the following week once swelling had subsided. Based on the radiographs showing a lateral malleolus fracture without signs of significant comminution, the plan was to proceed with open reduction and internal fixation with a lag screw and neutralization plate following the principles of absolute stability. The posterior malleolus fragment did not involve a significant portion of the articular surface and did not require internal fixation.

Surgical Tact

Positioning

The patient is positioned supine on a radiolucent operating room table with a radiolucent distal extension if available. A tightly rolled small bump is placed under the ipsilateral posterosuperior iliac spine to combat external rotation of the leg and allow for easier access to the lateral malleolus. A radiolucent foam ramp is placed under the ipsilateral extremity to aid in intraoperative imaging by positioning the operative extremity at a higher level than the contralateral limb (to allow for unimpeded lateral view), and the C-arm is placed on the contralateral side of the table.

Approach

The author prefers to use a posterolateral approach to the fibula, placing the incision along the posterior border of the fibula. Dissection is carried down to the fascia with care to protect any branches of the superficial peroneal nerve, although the more posterior placement of the incision usually keeps the nerve in the anterior skin flap and away from the surgical field. The peroneal tendons and muscles are retracted posteriorly and protected throughout the approach and procedure. Minimal retraction is performed to relieve tension on the soft tissues.

Fracture Reduction and Fixation

Following exposure and debridement of periosteum from the fracture site including sharp excision of any periosteum interposed within the fracture site, pointed reduction forceps are used to obtain an anatomic reduction of the fibula. Given the oblique nature of the fracture, and limited comminution, fixation is amenable to a lag screw. A 3.5 mm lag screw is then placed perpendicular to the fracture site in a lag-by-technique fashion, in an anterosuperior to posteroinferior direction. After placement of the 3.5 mm lag screw, a one-third tubular plate is pre-contoured and provisionally held to the lateral side of the fibula with reduction forceps. Fibular length, rotation, as well as appropriate plate placement and length are verified fluoroscopically on AP and lateral views. The plate is fixed proximally with 3.5 mm bicortical screws and distally with 4.0 mm unicortical fully threaded cancellous screws. After fixation of the fibula, an external rotation stress test was performed and showed widening of the medial clear space, so placement of a syndesmotic screw was required. With the ankle held in dorsiflexion, a large pointed reduction clamp was placed across the syndesmosis with one tine on the fibula and the second tine on the tibia just proximal to the medial malleolus through a small stab incision to obtain and maintain an adequate reduction of the syndesmosis on the mortise view. A quadricortical 3.5 mm cortical screw was then placed through the fibula, across the syndesmosis and into the tibia. Intraoperative fluoroscopic views showed acceptable reduction and fixation of the lateral malleolus and syndesmosis (Fig. 1.2). The wound was closed and the leg was placed in a short leg splint postoperatively.

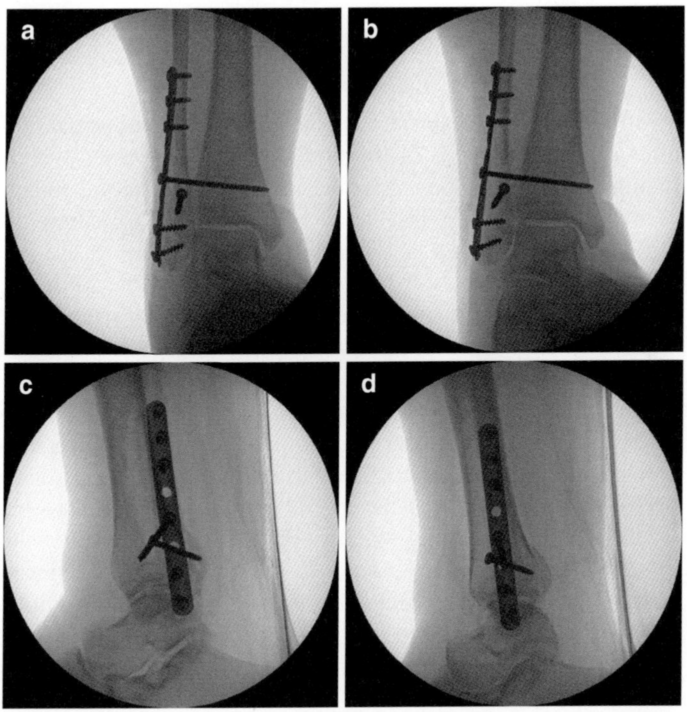

FIGURE 1.2 AP (**a**), mortise (**b**), and lateral (**c**) intraoperative fluoroscopic views showing lag-screw fixation of the lateral malleolus, and placement of a lateral neutralization plate and syndesmotic screw. A view parallel to the long axis of the syndesmotic screw (**d**) shows appropriate placement of the screw through both the fibula and the tibia

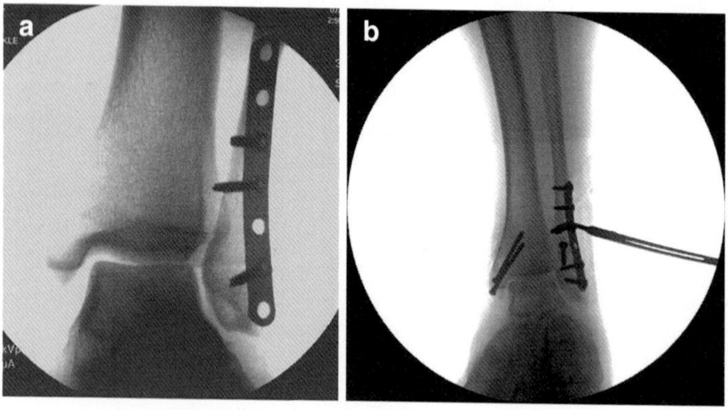

FIGURE 1.3 Intraoperative external rotation stress test (**a**) and Cotton test (**b**)

Stress testing to determine the need for syndesmotic fixation after rigid stabilization of the fibula can be performed with a manual external rotation stress test, or with direct lateral pulling of the fibula (Cotton Test), examples of which are shown in Fig. 1.3 in other patients. While the author prefers to use the manual external rotation test, either test is valuable to detect unstable syndesmotic injuries despite rigid malleolar fixation [5].

In terms of surgical technique for placement of syndesmotic screws, neither the number of screws (two vs. one) nor the size of the screws (3.5 mm vs. 4.5 mm cortical screws) makes a difference in clinical outcomes in compliant patients. This is also true for the number of cortices (tricortical vs. quadricortical) across which the screw is placed [6]. Although it is also possible to address the syndesmotic injury directly with fixation of the posterior malleolus, based on both the small size and comminution of the posterior malleolus fragment, trans-syndesmotic screw fixation was chosen for this particular fracture [6].

Postoperative Protocol

A short leg plaster splint was placed and the patient was to be non-weight bearing for a period of 6 weeks. Per the author's preference, at 2 weeks, sutures are removed and a removable boot is placed to allow range-of-motion exercises while the patient remains non-weight bearing. At 6 weeks, radiographs are obtained and the patient advanced to weight bearing as tolerated.

Outcome

The patient was followed for 1 year with regular radiographs. The 1-year postoperative radiographs shown in Fig. 1.4 demonstrate union of the lateral malleolus with no evidence of any hardware complications. Lucency is noted around the syndesmotic screw, but the screw itself remains intact. The mortise is intact in all views and there are no signs of degenerative changes in the tibiotalar joint. Clinically, the patient is able to dorsiflex to 20° and plantarflex to 45°. She ambulates with a normal gait without any assistive devices.

The author's preference is to avoid performing routine hardware removal. Syndesmotic screws as well as the lateral plate and screws are removed only if they become symptomatic. Retained screws do not significantly impair functional capacity, even in the syndesmosis, and retention of hardware is also more cost effective compared to elective screw

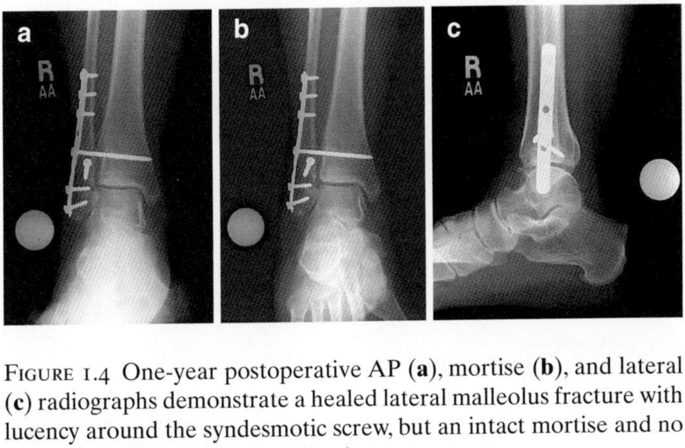

FIGURE 1.4 One-year postoperative AP (**a**), mortise (**b**), and lateral (**c**) radiographs demonstrate a healed lateral malleolus fracture with lucency around the syndesmotic screw, but an intact mortise and no evidence of posttraumatic arthrosis

removal. It is important to advise the patient early in the postoperative course that due to normal motion at the syndesmosis, the syndesmotic screw may show signs of loosening or even break but this has no clinical significance and does not indicate the need for additional surgery once the syndesmosis has healed.

Salient Points/Pearls

Lateral malleolus fractures with an associated medial deltoid ligament injury (SER IV) are unstable and require different management than an isolated lateral malleolus fracture.

- If injury radiographs do not demonstrate obvious medial clear space widening, it is important to obtain a stress radiograph to evaluate deltoid ligament competence.
- The presence of greater than 5 mm of medial clear space widening on a stress radiograph indicates an unstable injury pattern that is best managed with operative fixation.
- Once the fibula is stabilized intraoperatively, the stability of the syndesmosis needs to be assessed with either a Cotton test or an external rotation stress test to determine the need for syndesmosis fixation.
- The size of the screws, number of screws used, and number of cortices crossed (3 or 4) do not affect the outcome of syndesmotic fixation.
- Despite trends towards earlier weight bearing after operative fixation of ankle fracture, patients should be non-weight bearing for at least 6 weeks after syndesmotic fixation.
- A syndesmotic injury predicts a worse outcome than seen with lateral malleolus fractures that do not require syndesmotic fixation.

References

1. Ramsey PL, Hamilton W. Changes in tibiotalar area of contact caused by lateral talar shift. J Bone Joint Surg Am. 1976;58(3):356–7.

2. Park SS, Kubiak EN, Egol KA, Kummer F, Koval KJ. Stress radiographs after ankle fracture: the effect of ankle position and deltoid ligament status on medial clear space measurements. J Orthop Trauma. 2006;20(1):11–8.
3. Egol KA, Amirtharajah M, Tejwani NC, Capla EL, Koval KJ. Ankle stress test for predicting the need for surgical fixation of isolated fibular fractures. J Bone Joint Surg Am. 2004;86-A(11):2393–8.
4. Gill JB, Risko T, Raducan V, Grimes JS, Schutt RC Jr. Comparison of manual and gravity stress radiographs for the evaluation of supination-external rotation fibular fractures. J Bone Joint Surg Am. 2007;89(5):994–9.
5. Jenkinson RJ, Sanders DW, Macleod MD, Domonkos A, Lydestadt J. Intraoperative diagnosis of syndesmosis injuries in external rotation ankle fractures. J Orthop Trauma. 2005;19(9):604–9.
6. Hoiness P, Stromsoe K. Tricortical versus quadricortical syndesmosis fixation in ankle fractures: a prospective, randomized study comparing two methods of syndesmosis fixation. J Orthop Trauma. 2004;18(6):331–7.

Chapter 2
Unimalleolar Fractures: Medial Malleolus Only

Sunil M. Shahane and Nikhil A. Gokhale

Case Presentation

This is a 40-year-old female who sustained closed injury to ankle following a twisting injury. She was brought to the emergency room for evaluation and underwent placement into a splint.

Injury films (Fig. 2.1) (AP, mortise, and lateral views) revealed an isolated fracture of the medial malleolus with a vertical fracture line indicating a supination adduction type of injury. Suspicion of an intra-articular step prompted us to perform a CT scan which confirmed our suspicion.

Treatment and timing of surgery: Surgery was planned on the sixth day after swelling subsided. Plan was to elevate the depressed fragment and apply an antiglide plate over the medial malleolus.

S.M. Shahane, M.S. (Orth.), M.Ch. (Orth.) (✉)
Senior Orthopaedic Consultant, Orthopaedic and Trauma Surgery, Nanavati Super Speciality Hospital, Mumbai, Maharashtra 400056, India
e-mail: smshahane@gmail.com

N.A. Gokhale, M.S. (Orth.), M.R.C.S. (Ed.)
Registrar in Orthopaedics, Trauma and Orthopaedics, Kings Mill Hospital, Sherwood Forest Hospitals, NHS Foundation Trust, Sutton in Ashfield, Nottinghamshire NG17 4JL, UK

N.C. Tejwani (ed.), *Fractures of the Foot and Ankle*,
DOI 10.1007/978-3-319-60456-5_2,

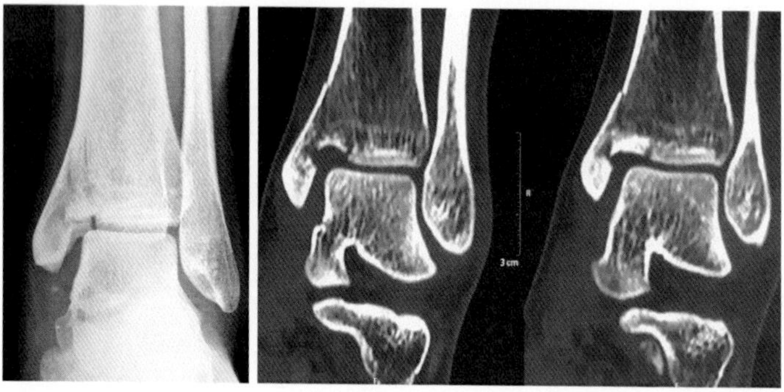

FIGURE 2.1 Anteroposterior X-ray post-injury and CT films showing intra-articular step

Surgical Tact

Position: Supine position under spinal anesthesia.

Approach: A J-shaped incision curving anteriorly (Fig. 2.2) was used over the medial malleolus to gain access to the medial malleolus and the anteromedial corner of the tibial plafond.

Fracture reduction and fixation: A small-incision arthrotomy was done in the anteromedial part of the tibial plafond to allow a small curved mosquito forceps to be passed in to feel for the depressed fragment. The depressed fragment was elevated through the fracture site under fluoroscopic guidance and the fracture was reduced using a clamp. K-wires were used to provisionally hold the reduction. Reduction was confirmed on fluoroscopy and by feeling for the depressed fragment using a curved mosquito forceps. A T-plate was used in antiglide mode for fixation with the lower screws acting as raft screws subchondrally (Fig. 2.3).

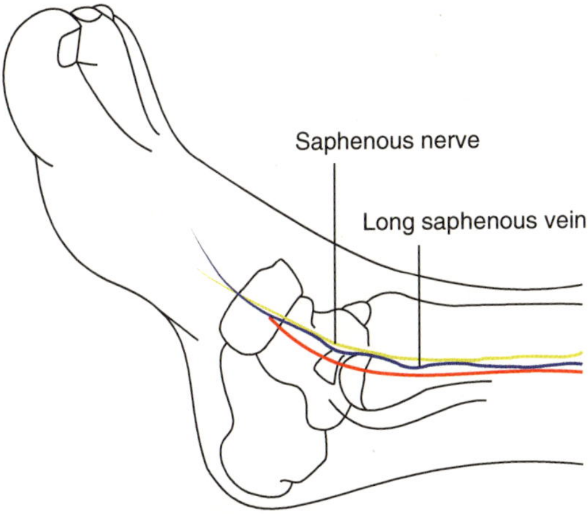

FIGURE 2.2 J-shaped skin incision curving anteriorly

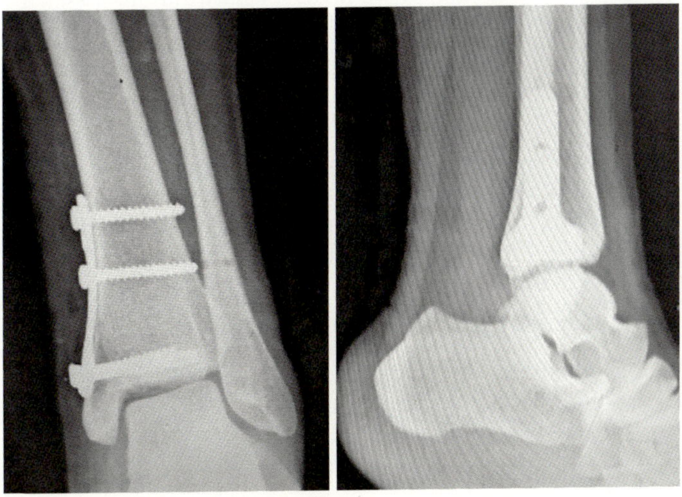

FIGURE 2.3 Postoperative X-rays

Postoperative Plan

A short leg splint was placed for 3 days for comfort and pain control. Range-of-motion exercises were started after 3 days. The patient remained non-weight bearing for 6 weeks after which partial weight bearing was started.

At 12 weeks, the patient was full weight bearing and had resumed household ambulation.

Outcome

Follow-up radiographs at 12 weeks show healed fracture. She had residual swelling which took another 6 weeks to disappear completely. Patient returned to full function at 6 months with full ankle motion.

Complications: None. No plans for hardware removal.

Salient Points/Pearls

- Herscovici in 2007 reported 57 isolated medial malleolus fractures and presented a classification system (Fig. 2.4). In his series, he obtained good results with conservative management of isolated medial malleolus fractures.

  Four simple patterns have been described:

  A—Tip avulsions
  B—Intermediate fracture line
  C—Fracture at the level of the plafond
  D—Fracture above the level of plafond

  The surgical management of a displaced medial malleolar fractures is often described in relation to its presentation as a part of bi- or tri-malleolar injuries. In such cases the recommendation is as follows:

  Type A fractures: These are avulsion fractures of the anterior colliculus. Surgery must be aimed at fixation of the avulsed fragment. Generally the avulsed fragment is small

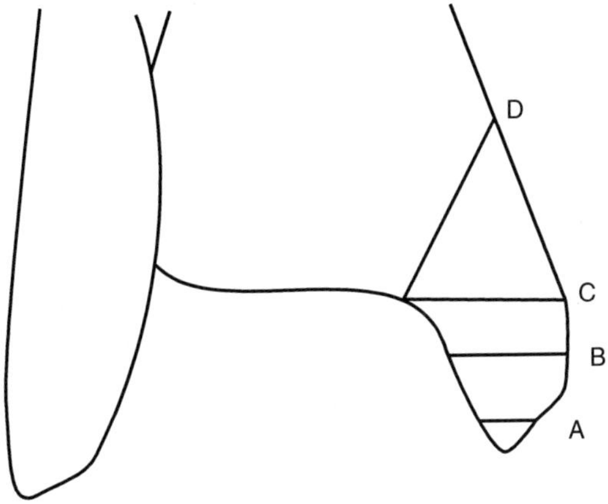

FIGURE 2.4 Classification of medial malleolar fractures

and needs to be fixed with two K-wires, supplemented with a tension band. After fixing the avulsed anterior colliculus, if there is displacement of the talus within the mortise indicating a rupture of the deep deltoid ligament, it should be repaired/reconstructed appropriately.

Type B and C fractures: These are avulsion injuries and should be fixed using compression screws (two if possible to prevent rotation) or tension band wiring depending on the size of fragment. Screws inserted posterior to the anterior colliculus place the posterior tibial tendon at significant risk for injury or abutment. Hence, the posterior tibial tendon should be directly visualized prior to the placement of screws in the medial malleolus when they are inserted posterior to the anterior colliculus.

Type D fractures: These fractures require accurate reduction of the plafond. If there is an impacted area it should be elevated. Bone graft can be used to fill in any void left after elevation. Fixation can be achieved by using cancellous lag screws perpendicular to the fracture site or by using antiglide plates.

- It is advisable to wait for the swelling to subside before operating on these fractures to reduce the chances of postoperative wound complications. It is also important to raise thick flaps.

- Care should be taken to avoid injury to the saphenous vein and nerve in the anterior aspect of the incision and the posterior tibial tendon in the distal aspect of the incision.
- Ankle range of motion should be started as soon as permissible to avoid postoperative ankle stiffness. Weight bearing is avoided till 6 weeks after surgery.

Further Reading

1. Davidovitch RI, Egol KA. The medial malleolus osteoligamentous complex and its role in ankle fractures. Bull NYU Hosp Jt Dis. 2009;67(4):318–324.
2. Pankovich AM, Shivraram MS. Anatomical basis of variability in injuries of the medial malleolus and the deltoid ligament. Acta Orthop Scand. 1979;50:217–223.
3. Herscovici D, Scaduto JM, Infante A. Conservative treatment of isolated fractures of the medial malleolus. J Bone Joint Surg Br. 2007;89(1):89–93.
4. Trauma and orthopaedic classifications: a comprehensive overview. In: Lasanianos NG, Kanakaris NK, Giannoudis PV, editors. Medial malleoli fractures. p. 371–3.
5. Femino JE, Gruber BF, Karunakar MA. Safe zone for the placement of medial malleolar screws. J Bone Joint Surg Am. 2007;89 (1):133–38.

Chapter 3
Bimalleolar Ankle Fracture: Medial Screws

Sanjit R. Konda

Case Presentation

A 52-year-old female with a past medical history of hypertension and hyperlipidemia was brought to the emergency room by ambulance after falling down two stairs. On physical examination her injury was isolated to her left ankle. She had a gross deformity about her ankle and no open wounds. She had a normal sensory and motor examination. Plain radiographs demonstrated a bimalleolar ankle fracture-dislocation. An intra-articular hematoma block was administered with 10 cc of 1% lidocaine to provide local anesthesia, a closed reduction was performed, and the patient was placed into a well-padded short leg plaster splint with a posterior slab and U-slab.

S.R. Konda, M.D.
Jamaica Hospital Medical Center, Queens, NY, USA

Department of Orthopaedic Surgery, NYU Langone Medical Center, NYU Hospital for Joint Diseases, New York, NY, USA
e-mail: Sanjit.konda@nyumc.org

N.C. Tejwani (ed.), *Fractures of the Foot and Ankle*,
DOI 10.1007/978-3-319-60456-5_3,

Injury and Post-reduction Films

AP, mortise, and lateral plain radiographs of the left ankle demonstrate a displaced short oblique fracture of the distal fibula at the level of the tibial plafond (Weber B) and a displaced transverse medial malleolar fracture. The talus is subluxed laterally on the AP and mortise view and posteriorly on the lateral view (Fig. 3.1). Post-reduction plain radiograph AP, mortise, and lateral views demonstrate that the talus is now reduced under the tibial plafond (Fig. 3.2).

Treatment and Timing of Surgery

In this patient because the ankle was reduced in an expeditious manner, there was minimal swelling about the ankle. Thus, the patient was able to be taken to the operating room the same day for operative fixation of her ankle. Had there been significant swelling about the ankle or a delay in closed reduction that would have predisposed the patient to significant swelling about the ankle, then delayed operative fixation would have been reasonable until the swelling subsided.

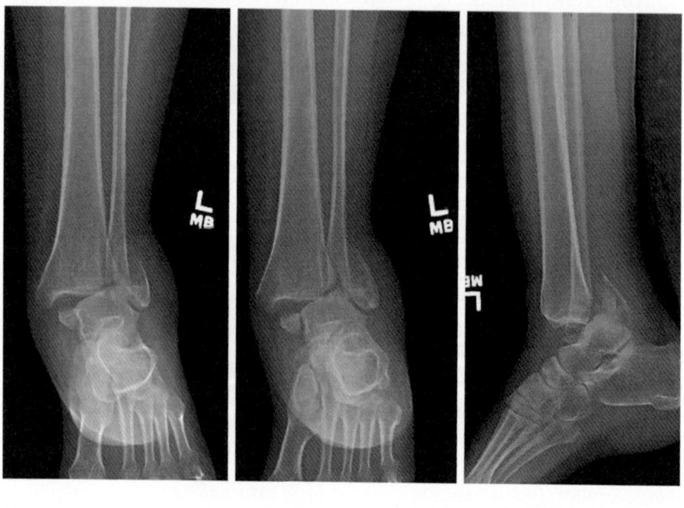

FIGURE 3.1 Injury films AP, mortise, and lateral

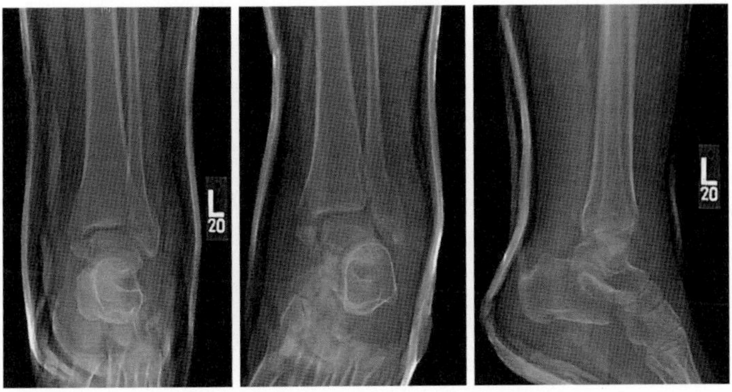

FIGURE 3.2 Post-reduction films AP, mortise, lateral

In terms of fixation strategy, the fracture pattern of the fibula was amenable to lag-screw fixation of the short oblique fibula fracture and neutralization of this screw with a laterally based plate adhering to principles of absolute stability fixation. Similarly, the transverse nature of the medial malleolar fracture was amenable to lag-screw fixation to compress the fracture also providing absolute stability.

Surgical Tact

Position

The patient is positioned supine on the operating room table with a small bump under the ipsilateral hip to internally rotate the leg such that the patella is pointing directly towards the ceiling. The leg is elevated off the table with a ramp of sheets placed under the thigh and tibia such that the knee is flexed 30° and the tibia remains parallel to the ground. A thigh tourniquet is utilized and is set to 100 mmHg above the systolic blood pressure (generally around 250 mmHg). The fluoroscopy machine is situated on the contralateral side of the injured extremity and the surgical implants and tools are situated on the ipsilateral side.

Approach: Medial Malleolus

A 4 cm incision centered over the medial malleolus and curved slightly anteriorly at the tip of the medial malleolus is used to expose the fracture site. Dissection is carried down to the fracture site with care taken to protect the saphenous vein and nerve.

Fracture Reduction and Fixation

After displacing the medial malleolus, removing any debris from the tibia-talar joint space, and clearing the fracture site of interposed clot and/or periosteum, fracture reduction is performed. First, a pilot hole is drilled with a 2.5 mm drill into the medial tibia 1 cm proximal to the fracture and in the midline of the fracture. A small pointed bone reduction clamp is then used to reduce the fracture anatomically with care taken to ensure that the visualized anterior and medial cortices of the fracture key in perfectly. After the fracture is reduced, fluoroscopic images are obtained to confirm the reduction.

Next, fracture fixation is performed; initially guide wires are inserted from the tip of the medial malleolus across the fracture under fluoroscopic control. Attention must be paid to the direction of the wires, such that they are parallel to each other and perpendicular to the fracture. Two 4.0 mm partially threaded non-cannulated cancellous screws are used for fixation. The screws are placed in parallel fashion and tightened sequentially to allow for increased compression at the fracture site while minimizing rotatory displacement. Care is taken to avoid too posterior placement of the screw on the medial malleolus as it can cause irritation on the posterior tibial tendon. Next, a stress examination of the ankle is performed to evaluate for distal syndesmotic injury and the syndesmosis is noted to be stable without widening. Final fluoroscopic XRs are obtained including AP, mortise, lateral, and a lateral external rotation view which confirm concentric reduction of the ankle mortise and anatomic reduction of the fibula and the medial malleolus (Fig. 3.3).

Postoperative Plan

The patient is placed into a well-padded short leg plaster splint with a posterior slab and U-slab. The patient is discharged home the same day with aspirin 325 mg as DVT prophylaxis. She is instructed to remain non-weight bearing for a total of 6 weeks postoperatively and to follow up in the office in 2 weeks for suture removal.

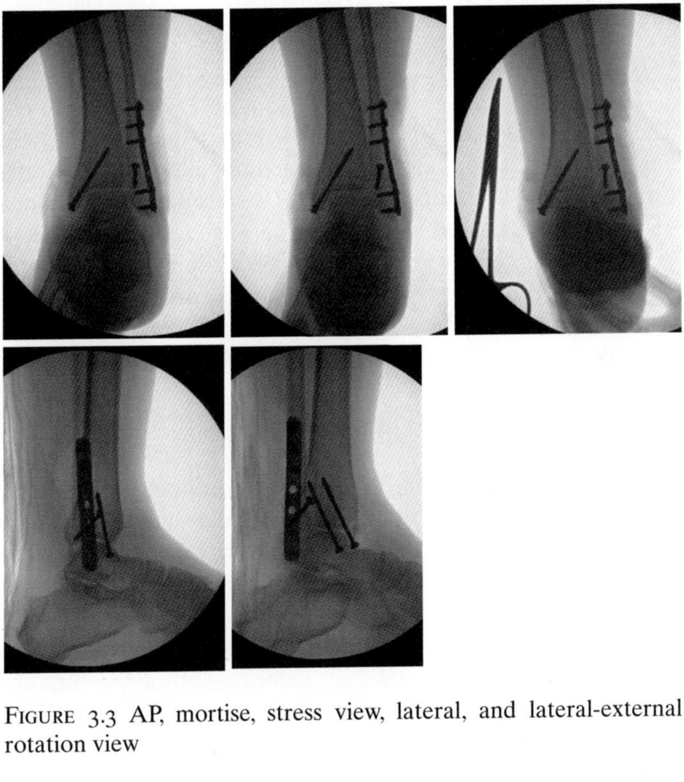

FIGURE 3.3 AP, mortise, stress view, lateral, and lateral-external rotation view

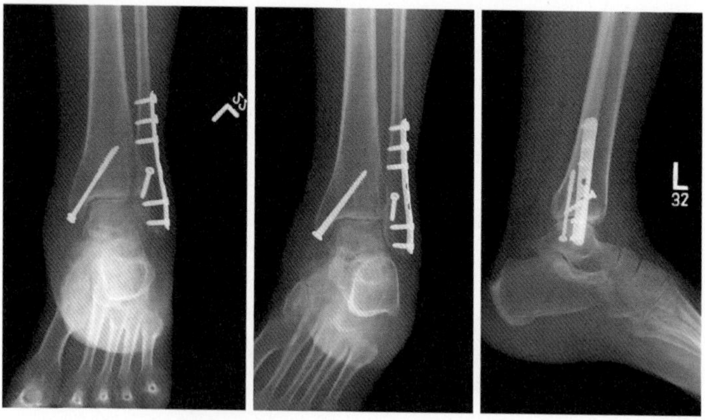

FIGURE 3.4 1-year postoperative radiographs: AP, mortise, and lateral

Outcome

The patient has been followed for 1 year postoperatively and her radiographs demonstrate a healed bimalleolar ankle fracture with consolidation at the fracture sites and maintenance of the concentric reduction of the ankle mortise (Fig. 3.4). She completed a short course of physical therapy and gradually returned to impact activities and is able to ambulate without an assistive device.

Salient Points/Pearls

- The medial malleolus confirms anterolateral rotational stability to the talus under the tibial plafond [1, 2].
- Transverse or short oblique fractures of the medial malleolus are amenable to lag by design fracture fixation using partially threaded cancellous screws.
- Comminuted fractures of the medial malleolus can be fixed with screw fixation; however, compression of the fracture should be avoided as this will lead to malreduction of the

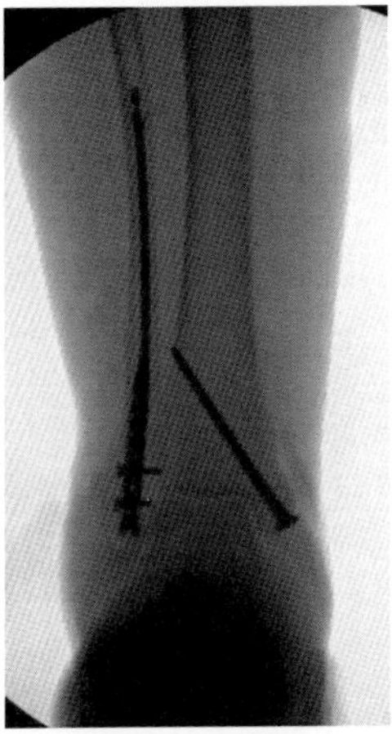

FIGURE 3.5 Bicortical medial malleolar screw fixation to prevent over-compression and displacement of the medial malleolar fracture

fracture. In this scenario, bicortical fully threaded screw fixation scan be used to serve as a strut to maintain the medial malleolar reduction (Fig. 3.5).

- Open reduction and internal fixation is recommended over percutaneous fixation of the fracture to achieve anatomic fracture reduction.
- In the setting of truly nondisplaced medial malleolar fracture that would benefit from operative fixation, percutaneous fixation can be achieved with cannulated 4.0 mm partially threaded screws.
- Placement of two screws (instead of one screw) is needed to avoid rotation of the medial malleolus fragment.
- Avoid placement of the medial malleolar screw in a position where the screw head will be in contact with the posterior tibial tendon as this can lead to chronic posterior tibial tendonitis.
- A lateral external rotation view of the medial malleolus can help judge medial malleolar reduction in an orthogonal plane to the ankle mortise radiographic view.

References

1. Michelson JD, Waldman B. An axially loaded model of the ankle after pronation external rotation injury. Clin Orthop Relat Res. 1996;328:285–93.
2. Davidovitch RI, Egol KA. The medial malleolus osteoligamentous complex and its role in ankle fractures. Bull NYU Hosp Jt Dis. 2009;67(4):318–24.

Chapter 4
Bimalleolar Ankle Fracture: Medial Plate

Marilyn Heng, Mitch Harris, and Michael J. Weaver

Clinical Scenario

A 37-year-old female presents to the emergency department with an isolated left-ankle injury. She slipped and fell going down her basement stairs and twisted her left ankle. She is a healthy woman with no significant medical history and she is a non-smoker.

On physical examination, the patient has swelling and tenderness of the left ankle. There is obvious deformity of the ankle but the skin is intact and non-threatened. Distal motor and sensory examination is intact.

Initial injury X-rays (Fig. 4.1) reveal a fracture-dislocation of the ankle consistent with a supination-adduction (SAD) mechanism per Lauge-Hansen classification [1]. A transverse

M. Heng, M.D., M.P.H., F.R.C.S.C.
Orthopaedic Surgery, Massachusetts General Hospital, Harvard Orthopaedic Trauma Initiative, Boston, MA 02114, USA

M. Harris, M.D. (✉) • M.J. Weaver, M.D.
Orthopaedic Surgery, Brigham and Women's Hospital, Boston, MA 02115, USA
e-mail: mbharris@partners.org

N.C. Tejwani (ed.), *Fractures of the Foot and Ankle*,
DOI 10.1007/978-3-319-60456-5_4,

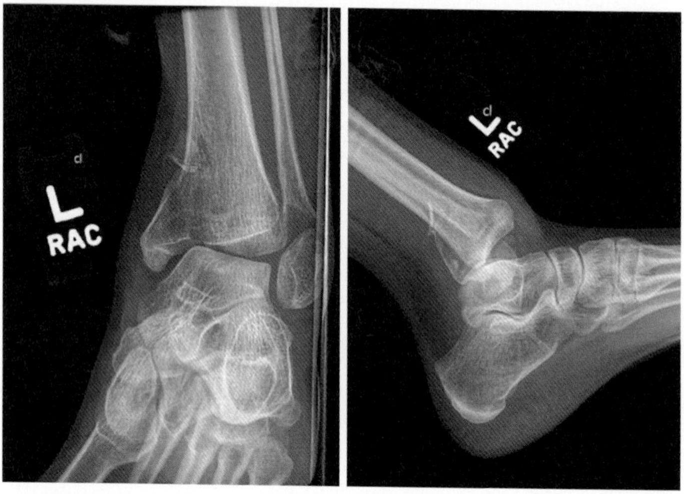

FIGURE 4.1 Initial injury AP and lateral radiographs

fibula fracture at the level of the mortise and a vertical medial malleolus fracture are the characteristic radiographic findings of an SAD-type ankle fracture.

The patient underwent closed reduction of the ankle under hematoma block, was placed into a plaster splint, and was scheduled for surgical management.

Treatment Considerations and Planning

The vertical nature of the medial malleolus fracture line lends itself well to fixation with an anti-glide/buttress construct. Usually, a one-third tubular plate is sufficient.

The classic sequence of events in a SAD ankle fracture involves the talus being driven medially against the medial malleolus (Fig. 4.2). This has the potential to cause marginal impaction at the medial tibial plafond [2]. A CT scan of the ankle is often useful in confirming the presence/absence of medial impaction at the articular surface (Fig. 4.3). The impaction may be located at the axilla of the medial plafond or on the medial aspect of the stable distal

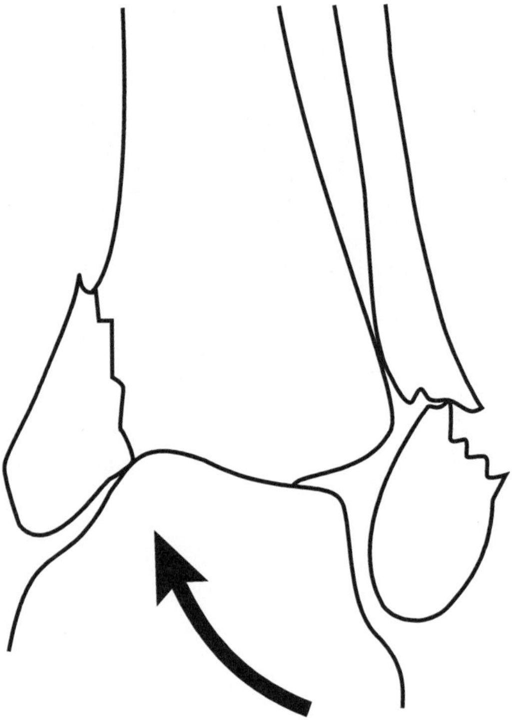

Figure 4.2 Supination-adduction fracture mechanism results in talus being driven medially into the axially of the medial malleolus

tibia articular surface (Fig. 4.4). It is important to recognize the marginal impaction in order to address and correct it at the time of surgery. A CT scan can also be useful in identifying the location of the apex of the medial fracture, allowing exact placement of the most optimal surgical incision (Fig. 4.5).

Surgical Timing

Most ankle fractures will allow for acute open reduction internal fixation. Delay in medial plating is recommended in instances of extreme significant swelling (without skin wrinkling),

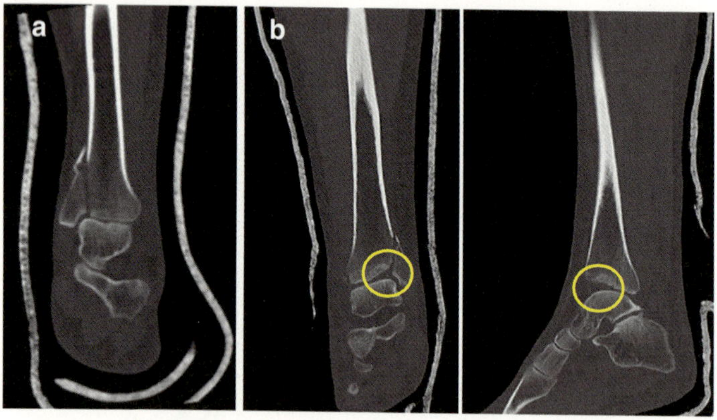

FIGURE 4.3 CT scan of the ankle demonstrating (**a**) absence of marginal impaction, (**b**) presence of marginal impaction (**note: **b** images are from different patient)

local abrasions associated with the injury or haemorrhagic blistering at the site of intended incision due to the concern for the inability to close the surgical incision, or subsequent wound healing and infection issues.

Surgical Tact

Position

The surgery is performed on a radiolucent table with a stack of blankets or a foam block used to create a platform to allow for acquisition of lateral imaging without lifting or manipulating the leg (Fig. 4.6). Patients should be positioned supine with a bump placed under the ipsilateral hip especially if the leg lies in significant external rotation at rest such that the foot points straight up and down. This allows for access to both the medial and lateral sides of the ankle. The authors prefer to use a tourniquet; however this is not mandatory.

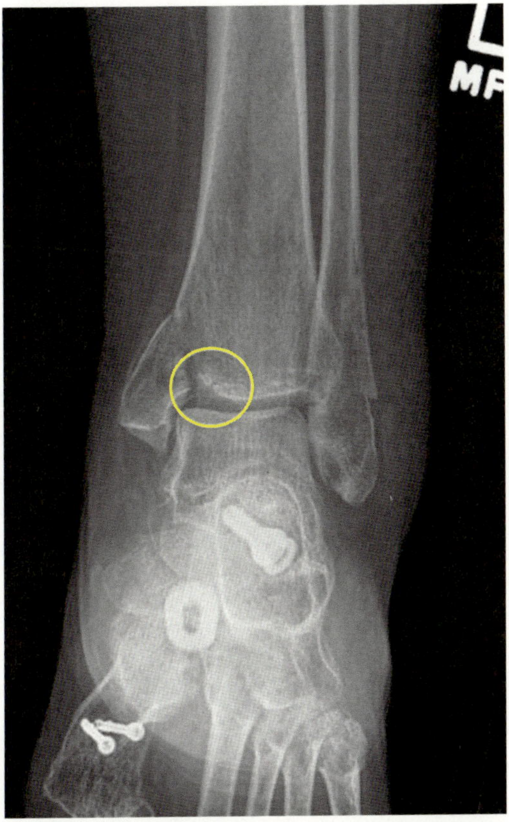

FIGURE 4.4 Marginal impaction seen on AP radiograph (** note: different patient from case example)

Approach

Careful evaluation of the CT scan can help with planning the medial surgical approach. It is important to plan an incision that will allow you to visualize the fracture line, and place a plate over the apex of the fracture to create a buttress. As many of these injuries involve articular impaction, visualization of this portion of the ankle joint to allow for reduction of

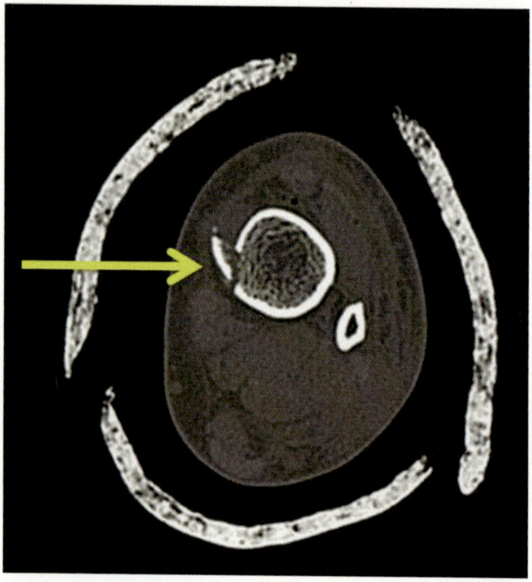

FIGURE 4.5 Identifying the apex (*yellow arrow*) of the medial fracture in order to plan the surgical approach

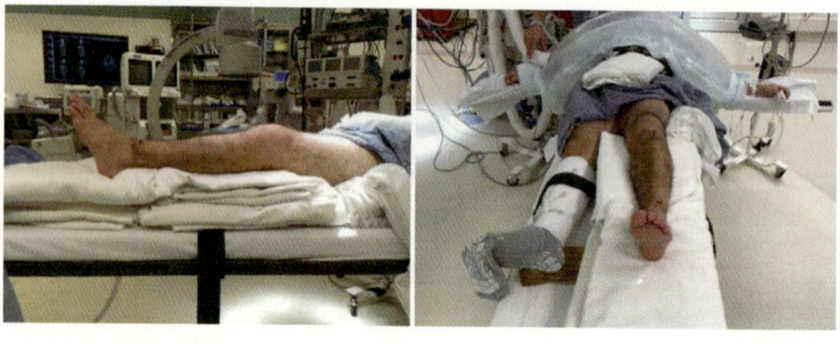

FIGURE 4.6 Setup and patient positioning for ankle fracture surgery

the joint surface and bone grafting or fixation is useful. Typically, an anteromedial incision permits adequate access to address these surgical goals.

Once the skin incision has been made, care should be taken to identify and protect the saphenous vein. Along the same course run the distal branches of the saphenous verve.

Injury to these small nerve branches can lead to a painful neuroma. Otherwise, apart from subcutaneous tissues, the exposure is taken directly down to bone. The apex of the fracture is identified and one can proceed with fracture reduction and fixation.

Fracture Reduction and Fixation

Supination adduction injuries involve medial translation of the talus. This impacts into the medial malleolus and causes fracture and displacement. The talus then subluxes medially. For this reason we find approaching the medial side of these injuries first to be helpful. As the fracture is reduced, and a buttress plate is applied, the talus reduces into the ankle mortise and an indirect reduction of the fibula occurs. This makes the eventual reduction and fixation of the fibula easier.

First the fracture is approached. Care is taken to avoid stripping periosteum from the bone beyond that needed to see and achieve the reduction. Often infolded periosteum and hematoma need to be debrided from within the fracture. A laminar spreader may then be used to book open the fracture to expose any areas of articular impaction.

Any impacted fragments are pushed back down into position. The talus can often be used as a mould to avoid over-reduction of the impacted articular portion. Once pushed down into position, the void left behind the fragments can be addressed. We typically use cancellous allograft chips either alone or mixed with demineralized bone matrix and vancomycin powder. Alternatively, calcium phosphate bone graft substitute can be used.

Once the articular surface of the tibial plafond has been addressed the medial malleolus fragment can be reduced into position. The provisional reduction can be maintained with small K-wires. A one-third tubular plate or other small fragment low-profile plate is selected and slightly under contoured to allow for a buttress effect. The plate is laid over the apex of the fracture and the proximal screws are placed first to compress the primary fracture line. Distal lag screws through the plate should be placed in order to apply compression across the fracture line.

C-arm fluoroscopy is used throughout to confirm an anatomic reduction of the joint surface and reduction of the ankle mortise and extra-articular placement of screws.

Once the medial side has been addressed attention can be turned to the fibula fracture. Unlike many ankle fractures, SAD patterns are associated with a transverse fracture pattern. This may be amenable to either plate fixation or occasionally an intramedullary screw/wire.

Closure

The wound is closed in layers. Given the high risk of wound complications with ankle fractures we prefer to use nylon sutures for the skin closure.

Post-operative Protocol

Post-operatively, the authors prefer to keep the patient in the plaster splint placed in the operating room at the end of surgery for 2 weeks. The patient is mobilized touch-down weight bearing on the affected leg. At 2-week follow-up, the leg is removed from the plaster splint and is allowed to begin active and passive range of motion of the ankle. The patient's weight-bearing restriction is lifted at 6 weeks post-operatively and the patient is encouraged to progress weight bearing as tolerated, first in an aircast boot and then weaning out of the boot when comfortable. Formal physical therapy is not necessarily required; however, certain patient populations may benefit, such as older patients for supervised guidance on gait training, ankle strengthening and proprioception, or athletes for sport-specific rehabilitation.

Follow-Up and Outcome

In general, patients are seen in follow-up at approximately 2 weeks, 6 weeks, and 3 months post-surgery. Weight bearing can begin between 6 and 12 weeks post-operatively depending on the degree of articular involvement and quality of the fixation. By 3 months post-operatively, our patient had returned to ambulating in regular shoes without the need for assistive ambulatory aid. She was pain free and her X-rays demonstrate good healing of the fracture (Fig. 4.7). She was discharged with instructions to gradually return to all of her activities and advised on the possibility for the need for hardware removal.

Fixation with a medial plate can result in irritation from the hardware, especially in thin patients. If required, symptomatic hardware can be removed after the fracture has completely healed typically after 9–12 months.

Outcomes of supination-adduction medial malleolus fractures treated with plating are good in the literature. In a case report of eight patients with associated marginal impaction,

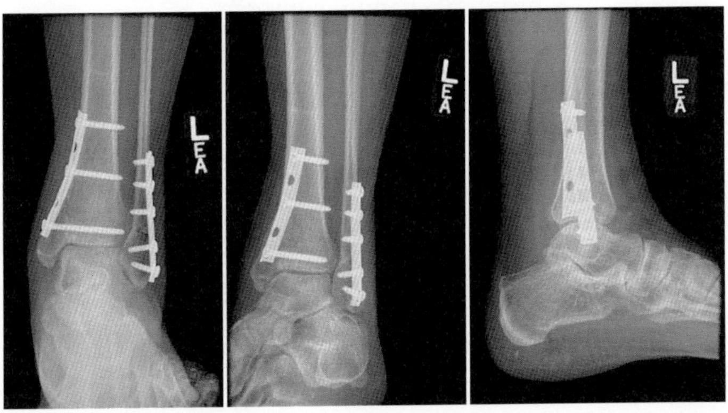

FIGURE 4.7 Final AP, mortise, and lateral radiographs of patient at 3-month follow-up

McConnell and Tornetta reported 100% union in 8 weeks, good-excellent clinical outcome scores, and one patient requiring screw removal [2]. More recently, Ebraheim et al. reported on six patients with vertical medial malleolus fractures treated with plating [3]. Ultimately all six patients achieved union with an average AOFAS score of 84 at 6 months post-operatively; however, the authors rated 17% of patient as having a delayed union.

Salient Points/Pearls

- Supination-adduction injuries often involve articular impaction. Obtain a CT scan to fully evaluate the articular surface and to locate the apex of the fracture to plan your surgical approach.
- Unlike most other ankle fracture types, in the case of a SAD fracture pattern, fixation of the tibia first may make the overall reduction easier, and often results in near-anatomic realignment and reduction of the fibula.
- During the medial approach, watch out for the saphenous vein and nerve. Although small, injury to the saphenous nerves may result in a painful neuroma.
- Reduction of the articular surface may require bone grafting or use of bone graft substitutes.

References

1. Lauge-Hansen N. Fractures of the ankle II. Combined experimental-surgical and experimental-roentgenologic investigations. Arch Surg. 1950;60(5):957–85.
2. McConnell T, Tornetta P. Marginal plafond impaction in association with supination-adduction ankle fractures: a report of eight cases. J Orthop Trauma. 2001;15(6):447–9.
3. Ebraheim NA, Ludwig T, Weston JT, Carroll T, Liu J. Comparison of surgical techniques of 111 medial malleolar fractures classified by fracture geometry. Foot Ankle Surg. 2014;20(4):276–80.

Chapter 5
Trimalleolar Ankle Fracture: Posterior Plate for Posterior Malleolus Fractures

Roy I. Davidovitch and Alexander M. Crespo

Introduction

Trimalleolar ankle fractures with a posterior malleolus component are low-energy injuries in which the posterior articular surface of the tibia is avulsed by the posteroinferior tibiofibular ligament. The indications for fixation of small nonarticular fractures are a matter of debate; however fixation of larger fragments associated with posterior instability of the mortise and articular incongruity is well established.

Case Presentation

Patient is a 29-year-old female presenting to the emergency ward status post a trip and fall incident with an isolated injury to the right ankle. Her skin was intact, and pulses were present

R.I. Davidovitch, M.D. (✉) • A.M. Crespo, M.D.
Orthopedic Surgery, NYU Hospital for Joint Diseases, New York, NY 10003, USA
e-mail: roy.davidovitch@nyumc.org

N.C. Tejwani (ed.), *Fractures of the Foot and Ankle*,
DOI 10.1007/978-3-319-60456-5_5,

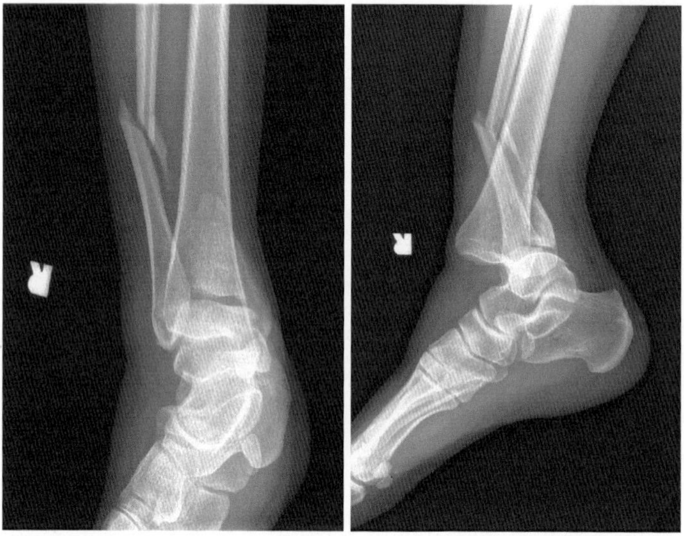

FIGURE 5.1 Initial radiographs demonstrating right trimalleolar fracture-dislocation

and symmetric. She had significant swelling and an obvious deformity of the ankle. Neurovascularly she was intact. Initial imagin.g revealed an isolated right trimalleolar fracture/dislocation (Fig. 5.1). She was indicated for conscious sedation and immediate closed reduction in the emergency ward (Fig. 5.2) to be followed by an ORIF procedure following admission.

Treatment Consideration

When obtaining the patient's history, it is important to address medical comorbidities and social habits that will influence the choice for operative intervention and postoperative management. Diabetic patients should undergo detailed peripheral vascular and neurologic examination. Signs of poor microvascular status and/or a history of smoking may prompt the surgeon toward less invasive fixation of

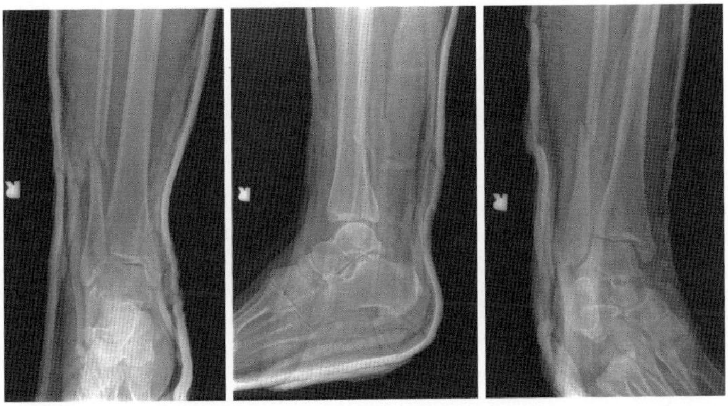

FIGURE 5.2 Post-reduction radiographs

posterior fragments (percutaneous screws) or nonoperative management due to the increased risk for wound complications. Presence of peripheral neuropathy warrants a prolonged period of non-weight bearing to minimize the risk of implant failure.

Standard X-rays of the ankle should always be obtained. The lateral X-ray is most important in determining the presence and nature of a posterior malleolus fracture. Posterior subluxation of the talus, signifying ligamentous instability, can be reliably identified on the lateral X-ray. If ambiguity exists it may be appropriate to obtain a CT scan of the ankle to better delineate the size of fracture fragment and possible articular comminution or impaction.

Historically, the most common indication for fixing the posterior malleolus has been for fragments greater than 25% of the articular surface [1, 2]. However, articular incongruity with greater than 2 mm step-off [3], syndesmotic associated instability [4, 5], and persistent posterior subluxation despite fibular fixation [6] has also been reported as indications for fixation. One study has shown that the syndesmosis is restored to 70% stability with isolated plating of the posterior malleolus versus only 40% stability restored with isolated syndesmotic fixation in the presence of PM fracture [5].

Operative Technique

The posterolateral approach to the ankle is the workhorse for internal fixation as this approach allows fixation of the posterior malleolus fragment as well as the fibula through a single incision [6, 7]. The patient is positioned prone on a radiolucent table (Fig. 5.3). An incision is made in the intermuscular plane between flexor hallucis longus and the peroneal tendons (Fig. 5.4). It is important to identify and preserve the sural nerve located in the subdermal fat layer, as this structure enters the surgical field in approximately 80% of cases [8]. It is our preference to always address the posterior malleolus fragment first as this can aid in restoring length to the fractured fibula. The periosteum is then elevated off the posterior tibia. The posterior malleolus is visualized with medial retraction of the FHL. If medial extension is present, it can sometimes be addressed with further medial retraction of the FHL although this pattern may be better addressed using the posteromedial approach. The fracture is mobilized from medial to lateral and proximal to distal to maintain the ligamentous attachment to the fragment [6]. The fracture fragment is booked open and hematoma is irrigated from

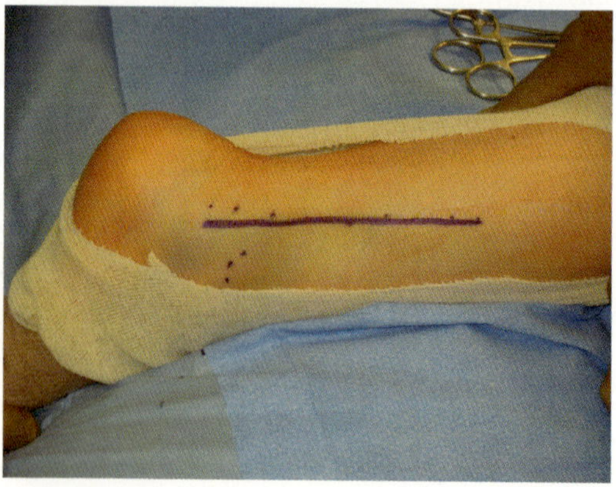

FIGURE 5.3 Patient positioned prone on radiolucent table

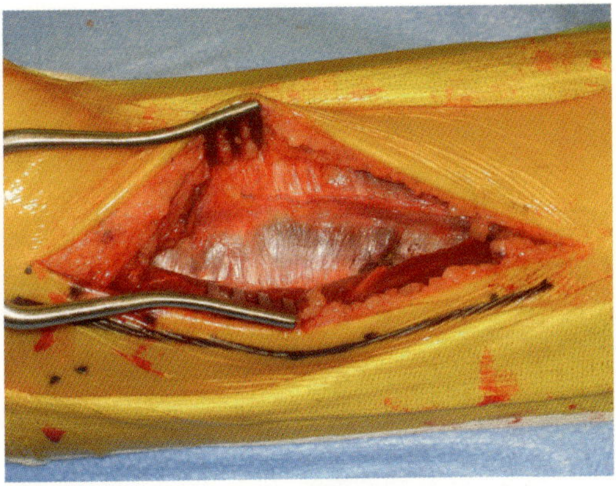

FIGURE 5.4 Posterolateral approach to the ankle

within the fracture to remove clot and any loose fragments of bone or tissue which may impede reduction. Reduction can be achieved using a variety of techniques although our preference is for gentle pressure using a ballpoint pusher device. A K-wire placed from posterior to anterior can aid in holding the reduction. Once this provisional reduction is obtained, a buttress plate with screw placement at the apex of the fracture is applied to prevent posterosuperior migration of the fragment. Additional 1–2 screws are placed proximal to the fracture after at least one lag screw is placed through the distal aspect of the plate in order to obtain compression across the fracture. The fibula may be addressed by either medial or lateral retraction of the peroneals and fixation achieved using a 1/3 tubular plate (Fig. 5.5). A stress view to assess the syndesmosis is performed at this point. In this case fixation of the posterior malleolus and fibula sufficiently stabilized the syndesmosis and transsyndesmotic fixation was not needed.

Options for fixing the posterior malleolus fragment include a standard 1/3 tubular plate for large noncomminuted fragments or a T-plate. Pre-contoured locked T-plates for the posterior malleolus are now available although we have not found them necessary in these cases. A displaced medial

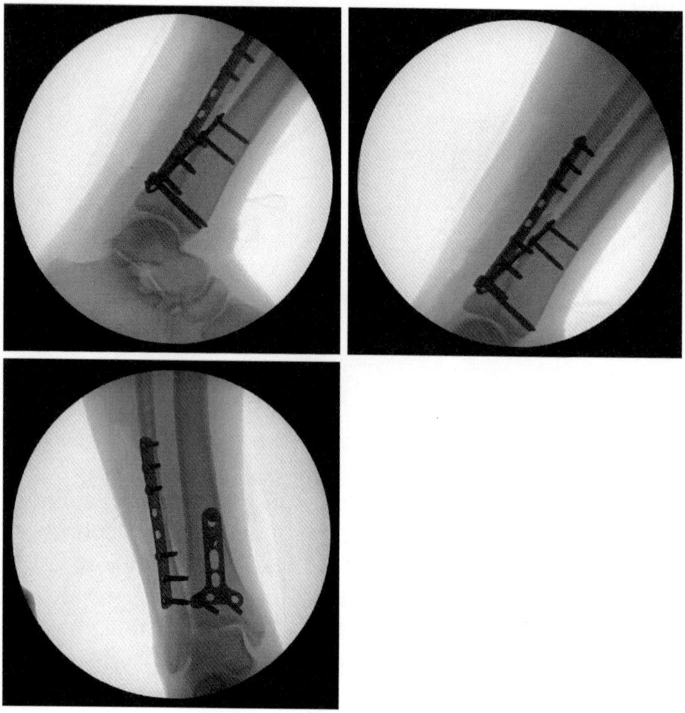

FIGURE 5.5 Fixation of the posterior malleolus utilizing a 1/3rd tubular plate

malleolus fracture that requires fixation presents somewhat of a challenge with the patient in a prone position; however by internally rotating the entire lower extremity and utilizing a sterile bump to elevate the ankle the medial malleolus can be approached using a standard medial incision and the fracture repaired in standard fashion.

Post-op Care

It is our practice to immobilize the ankle in a short leg splint for 2 weeks postoperatively. We recommend a 6-week non-weight-bearing protocol for patients; however we encourage active and passive range of motion of the ankle as soon as 2 weeks at which point the splint is removed and removable walking boot is placed. Patients are seen again at 6 weeks where X-rays are obtained and upon signs of healing patients are allowed to weight bear as tolerated without a brace. Patients with a history of peripheral neuropathy are maintained non-weight bearing for a period of 12 weeks.

Outcomes

The patient followed the standard postoperative protocol as delineated above and healed uneventfully (Fig. 5.6). Patient was allowed to return to full activity including sports at 6 months.

Salient Points/Pearls

- The posterior malleolus is an important component of the distal tibia providing concentric articulation of the tibiotalar joint and attachment of the PITFL.
- Posterior malleolus fractures are heterogeneous in presentation and may range from small posterior lip avulsions to

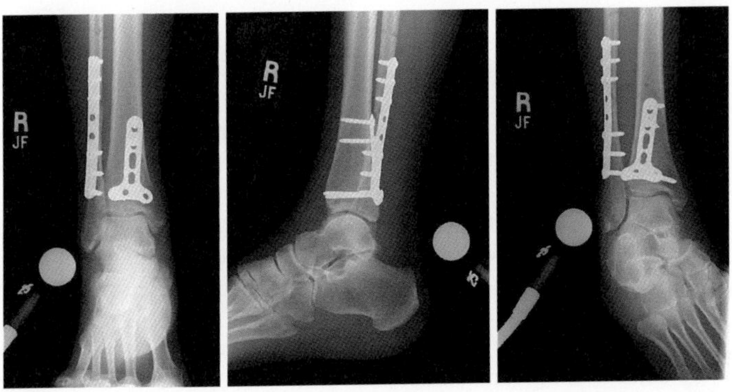

FIGURE 5.6 Radiographs demonstrating a healed trimalleolar fracture

large fragments comprising 50% or more of the articular surface. As a result, their capacity to impact articular congruity and syndesmotic stability is variable.

- Cross-sectional imaging of the ankle is useful in fully characterizing the posterior malleolus fragment size and identifying comminution; however often it is not necessary and X-ray images are sufficient. Fragments greater than or equal to 25% of the articular surface are commonly indicated for surgery, although this rule of thumb is not clearly proven and should not serve as an absolute indication.
- It is important to consider other factors such as articular congruity and ankle stability when deciding whether to fix the PM fragment.
- Ultimately, the presence of a posterior malleolus fracture appears to portend a worse clinical outcome and results of surgical intervention are varied.
- A posterolateral approach in lateral or prone (if associated medial fracture) position is useful to approach the back of the ankle.
- Fixation using a T-plate as buttress is recommended.
- The fibula is then fixed and finally the medial malleolus.
- Nonetheless, there is sufficient evidence to support plate fixation of posterior malleolus to restore articular congruity and syndesmotic stability which are likely the most important predictors of a successful outcome.

References

1. De Vries JS, Wijgman AJ, Siercvelt IN, Schaap GR. Long-term results of ankle fractures with a posterior malleolar fragment. J Foot Ankle Surg. 2005;44(3):211–7.
2. White TO, Bugler KE. Ankle fractures. In: Court-Brown CM, Heckman JD, MM MQ, et al., editors. Rockwood and Green's fractures in adults. Alphen aan den Rijn: Wolters Kluwer Health; 2014. p. 2542–91.
3. Berkes MB, Little MT, Lazaro LE. Articular congruity is associated with short-term clinical outcomes of operatively treated SER IV ankle fractures. J Bone Joint Surg Am. 2013;95(19):1769–75.

4. Gardner MJ, Brodsky A, Briggs SM, Nielson JH, Lorich DG. Fixation of posterior malleolar fractures provides greater syndesmotic stability. Clin Orthop Relat Res. 2006;447:165–71.
5. Gardner MJ, Demetrakopoulos D, Briggs SM, et al. Malreduction of the tibiofibular syndesmosis in ankle fractures. Foot Ankle Int. 2006;27(10):788–92.
6. Irwin TA, Lien J, Kadakia AR. Posterior malleolus fracture. J Am Acad Orthop Surg. 2013;21(1):32–40.
7. Abdelgawad AA, Kadous A, Kanlic E. Posterolateral approach for treatment of posterior malleolus fracture of the ankle. Foot Ankle Int. 2001;50:607–11.
8. Jowett AJ, Sheikh FT, Carare RO, et al. Location of the sural nerve during posterolateral approach to the ankle. Foot Ankle Int. 2010;31(10):880–3.

Chapter 6
Trimalleolar Ankle Fracture: Screws Only for Posterior Malleolus

Tonya L. Dixon, Brendan R. Southam, and Michael T. Archdeacon

Case Presentation

The patient is a 55-year-old female with a past medical history of depression and psychiatric illness who presented to the emergency department with right ankle pain after slipping in the mud after an altercation.

Obtained radiographic images revealed a trimalleolar ankle fracture dislocation (Figs. 6.1 and 6.2). The patient underwent closed reduction in the emergency room under conscious sedation and was admitted to the orthopedic service for definitive management.

T.L. Dixon, M.D., M.P.H. (✉)
Department of Orthopaedic Surgery, Division of Foot and Ankle Surgery, Massachusetts General Hospital, Waltham, MA, USA
e-mail: tonyaldixon@gmail.com

B.R. Southam, M.D. • M.T. Archdeacon, M.D., M.S.E.
Department of Orthopaedic Surgery, University of Cincinnati Academic Health Center, Cincinnati, OH, USA

N.C. Tejwani (ed.), *Fractures of the Foot and Ankle*,
DOI 10.1007/978-3-319-60456-5_6,

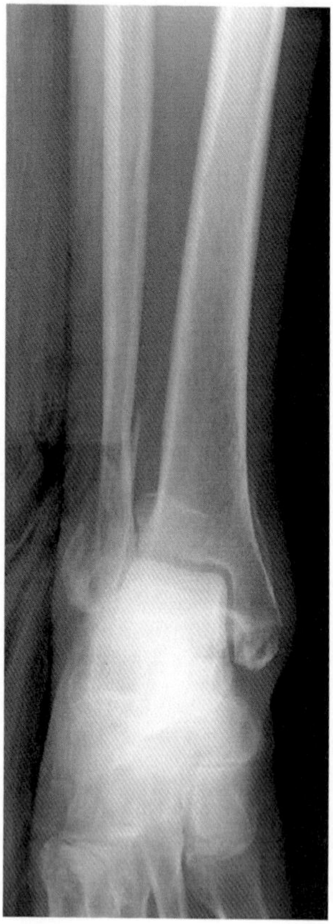

Figure 6.1 AP radiograph shows a trimalleolar ankle fracture

Treatment Considerations/Planning/Tests Needed

Ankle fractures are a common orthopedic injury, but more recent data suggest that reduction and fixation of the posterior malleolus is more critical than previously thought [1–4]. Previous literature supported that a posterior malleolar fragment of less than 25% of the articular surface would spontaneously reduce with the reduction and fixation of the lateral

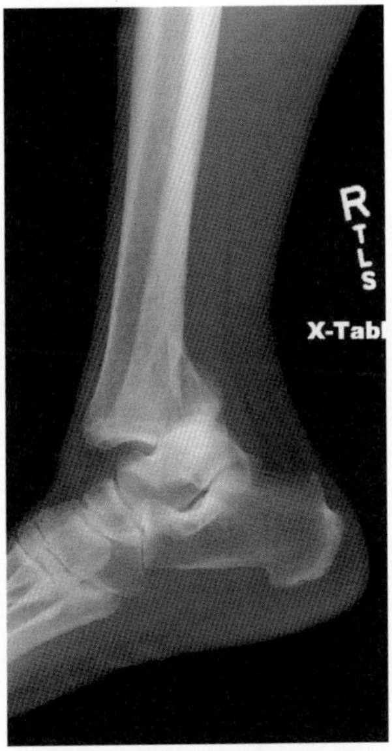

FIGURE 6.2 Lateral radiograph shows a dislocated tibiotalar joint with a sizeable posterior malleolus fracture fragment

malleolus, provided the posterior-inferior tibiofibular ligament is intact [1–6]. Odak et al. recommended that the posterior malleolus be fixed if it was associated with a fracture dislocation and intraoperative evaluation demonstrated the tibiotalar joint was not congruent or residual talar subluxation was present [3].

The decision to open reduce and fixate the posterior malleolus may be made in the operating room; thus, the surgeon should plan accordingly and have all possible equipment and implants available. It may be beneficial to obtain a computed tomography (CT) scan prior to surgical intervention to assess for impaction, determine fragment size, and assess incarcerated fragments that could inhibit reduction.

A contraindication to acute surgical fixation may be extensive soft tissue injury including hemorrhagic fracture blisters and compromised skin. A tenuous soft tissue envelope may require provisional external fixation to allow for evaluation and care of the soft tissues, as well as provide stability prior to definitive surgical intervention.

Timing of Surgery

The risk and benefits of the procedure were discussed with the patient, including nonoperative treatment. The patient elected to have surgical intervention and this was scheduled for the day following the injury given that her soft tissues were amenable to surgical intervention. In the event that she had excessive edema or fracture blisters, she would have remained in her splint with early follow-up to reassess the soft tissue envelope. If her ankle was unstable and difficult to keep reduced in the splint, provisional external fixation would be utilized until the soft tissues were amenable to surgical intervention. Typically, this occurs with some resolution of the edema and return of skin wrinkles around the foot and ankle.

Intraoperative Tips and Tricks for Reduction/Fixation

Position

Supine with a large bump or bean bag under the ipsilateral buttock to allow posterior access to the ankle if needed.

Approach

Standard direct lateral approach over the fibula. Dissect soft tissues down until you are directly on the bone. Care should be taken to protect the superficial peroneal (nerve located approx. 7 cm proximal to the tip of the fibula) if it is encountered during your dissection.

Fracture Reduction

The fibula is typically reduced with a pointed reduction clamp (Weber) and fixed with a lag screw when possible. We prefer a 2.7 mm lag screw (inserted A-P) when available, as the smaller profile is less likely to interfere with plate fixation. We then neutralize the construct with a lateral plate on the fibula, usually with a minimum of three screws proximal to the fracture, and three distal, when possible. In comminuted fractures or osteoporotic bone, an anatomic precontoured locking fibular plate can be helpful. This will vary depending on the fracture type as well as the degree of comminution.

After the lateral malleolus has been stabilized, reduction of the posterior malleolus is assessed using fluoroscopy. If the posterior malleolus is anatomically reduced with reduction of the fibula, it can be stabilized with percutaneous lag screws placed anterior to posterior. If the reduction of the posterior malleolus is not acceptable, a percutaneous reduction with a pointed reduction or periarticular clamp should be attempted. This can be facilitated by dorsiflexing the ankle and levering the talus against the anterior joint surface; thus, applying a tensile reduction force on the posterior malleolar fragment. If a percutaneous reduction is not successful, then an open approach is required.

At this point, we generally dissect on the posterior aspect of the peroneal tendons with care taken to avoid detaching the posterior tibiofibular ligament. With this exposure, the fracture can be cleaned and reduced under direct visualization, again with a pointed reduction or periarticular clamp. Once acceptable reduction is achieved, the fragment is stabilized with anterior to posterior lag screws. We prefer 3.5 mm screws as there is adequate space for slightly larger screws. Alternatively, 4.0 mm cancellous screws can be utilized, and cannulated screws are a reasonable option, particularly if provisional fixation with K-wires provides an appropriate trajectory for internal fixation. These screws are placed percutaneously with a small incision on the anterior tibia and blunt dissection to bone to avoid the neurovascular bundle and extensor tendons. Stabilization of the posterior malleolus could be performed with posterior-to-anterior screws which theoretically would be biomechanically advantageous given the screw head would provide compression rather than the screw thread. However, in our experience this can be difficult in the supine or sloppy lateral position, and care must be exercised to avoid damaging the neurovascular bundle or Achilles tendon.

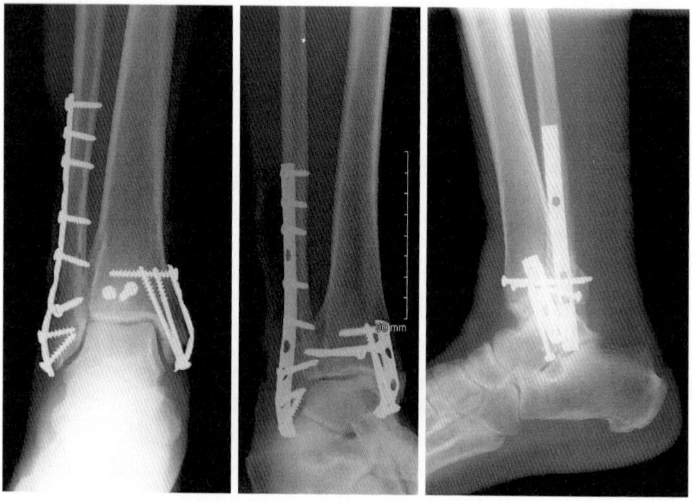

FIGURE 6.3 AP/Lateral/Oblique: Healed trimalleolar ankle fracture status post open reduction and internal fixation

Once fixation of the posterior malleolus has been achieved, attention is then directed to the medial malleolus. We prefer a direct medial incision centered over the fracture; however, a curvilinear incision toward the anterior-medial joint is very reasonable as well. Dissection to the fracture is performed with debridement of the hematoma and periosteum to facilitate reduction. The medial malleolar fragment is reduced with a pointed reduction clamp or a dental pick and provisionally stabilized with Kirschner wires. Fixation is completed with one or two lag screws or with a medial buttress plate. Final radiographic imaging confirms the reduction and the stability of fixation (Fig. 6.3). This is followed by wound closure and splinting with a well-padded sugar-tong and posterior splint in the neutral position.

Postoperative Plan

In general, the patient returns at 10–14 days for suture removal and follow-up radiographs. The patient is transitioned into a cast or removable boot while maintaining a non-weight bearing gait for a period of 6–12 weeks, depending on fracture stability and healing capacity. A diabetic patient should expect to be non-weight bearing for a minimum of 12 weeks before advancing their weight bearing status. Patients are seen in clinic every 6 weeks for clinical and radiographic evaluation until fracture healing occurs. Physical therapy is only prescribed for individuals who demonstrate needed assistance with regaining their strength and range of motion, or for more senior patients who need assistance with gait training and balance.

Outcome

The index patient remained non-weight bearing for a total of 12 weeks and transitioned into a walking boot with progressive weight bearing. The patient did not participate in formal physical therapy, and returned to full activities without restrictions. At 6 months after the initial injury, the patient returned to the operating room for elective removal of symptomatic, prominent hardware (Fig. 6.4). The patient had no further sequelae.

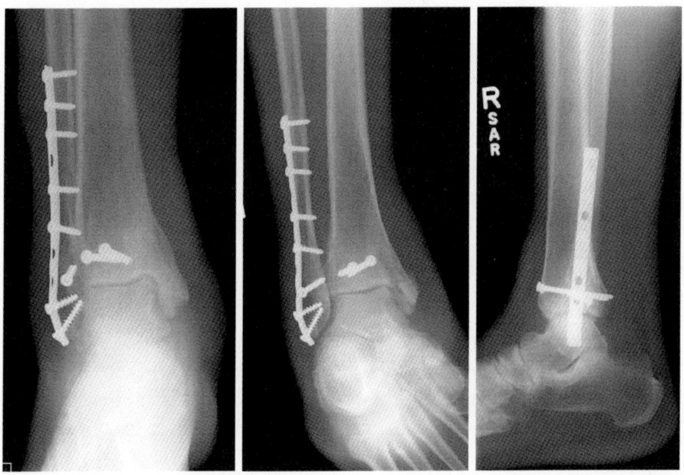

FIGURE 6.4 AP/Lateral/Oblique: Status post removal of symptomatic medial hardware

Salient Points/Pearls

- Timing of the surgical intervention is dictated by the soft tissue envelope.
- Reduction of the posterior malleolus can be achieved with closed, percutaneous or open reduction. A variety of reduction tools, including bone hook and pointed reduction clamps, with ankle manipulation can help with anatomic reduction.
- Fixation for the posterior malleolus is typically in the form of percutaneous lag screws placed anterior to posterior.
- Nearly full functional recovery should be expected in the majority of cases where an anatomic reduction is achieved.

References

1. Erdem MN, Erken HY, Burc H, Saka G, Korkmaz MF, Aydogan M. Comparison of lag screw versus buttress plate fixation of posterior malleolar fractures. Foot Ankle Int. 2014;35(10):1022–30. doi:10.1177/1071100714540893.
2. Mingo-Robinet J, Lopez-Duran L, Galeote JE, Martinez-Cervell C. Ankle fractures with posterior malleolar fragment: management and results. J Foot Ankle Surg. 2011;50:141–5. doi:10.1053/j.jfas.2010.12.013.
3. Odak S, Ahluwalia R, Unnikrishnan P, Hennessy M, Platt S. Management of posterior malleolar fractures: a systematic review. J Foot Ankle Surg. 2016;55:140–5. doi:10.1053/j.jfas.2015.04.001.
4. O'Connor TJ, Mueller B, Ly TV, Jacobson AR, Nelson ER, Cole PA. "A to P" screw versus posterolateral plate for posterior malleolus fixation in trimalleolar ankle fractures. J Trauma. 2015;29:e151–6.
5. Talbot M, Steenblock TR, Cole PA. Surgical technique: posterolateral approach for open reduction and internal fixation of trimalleolar ankle fractures. Can J Surg. 2005;48(6):487–90.
6. Franzone JM, Vosseller JT. Posterolateral approach for open reduction and internal fixation of a posterior malleolus fracture—hinging on an intact PITFL to disimpact the tibial plafond: a technical note. Foot Ankle Int. 2013;34(8):1177–81. doi:10.1177/1071100713481455.

Chapter 7
Maisonneuve Ankle Injuries

William Min

Case Presentation

This is a 37-year-old male patient without significant past medical history who sustained a twisting injury to his left lower extremity while playing soccer. He reports that he was planting his leg while trying to pivot into another direction, and felt pain about the ankle. He denies any other injuries. He localizes the pain along the affected lower extremity; it is centered over the ankle, but also is present diffusely about the length of the lower leg. He reports that he is unable to weight bear to the affected extremity.

On examination, the leg is diffusely swollen. There are no open injuries. He has tenderness primarily over the medial ankle and the anterolateral aspect of the ankle. There is also diffuse tenderness along the length of the leg,

W. Min, M.D., M.S., M.B.A.
The Hughston Clinic at Gwinnett Medical Center,
Lawrenceville, GA, USA
e-mail: min.william@gmail.com

N.C. Tejwani (ed.), *Fractures of the Foot and Ankle*,
DOI 10.1007/978-3-319-60456-5_7,

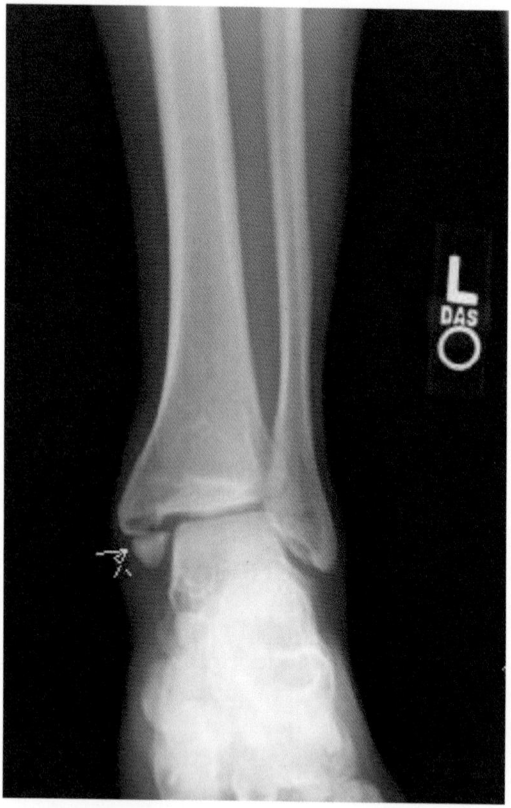

FIGURE 7.1 AP radiograph of the left ankle, revealing a displaced medial malleolus fracture

primarily along the anterior and lateral lower leg. Compartments are soft, and his neurovascular status is intact. His range of motion is limited due to pain. He has a positive squeeze test.

Imaging examinations of the ankle revealed a medial malleolus fracture (Figs. 7.1 and 7.2). However, given the above clinical examination, a tibia/fibula radiographic series was obtained, which revealed a proximal oblique fibular fracture (Figs. 7.3 and 7.4).

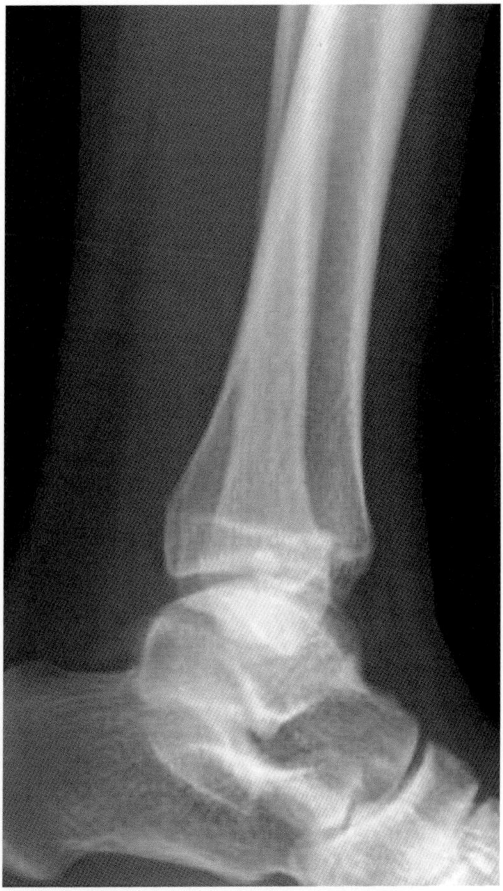

FIGURE 7.2 Lateral radiograph of the left ankle, revealing a displaced medial malleolus fracture

Given the above findings, the patient was diagnosed with a Maissoneuve fracture. He was recommended for operative stabilization of his injury, given the inherent instability of the ankle joint and the risks of mortise instability. Risks and benefits were discussed with the patient, and informed consent was obtained.

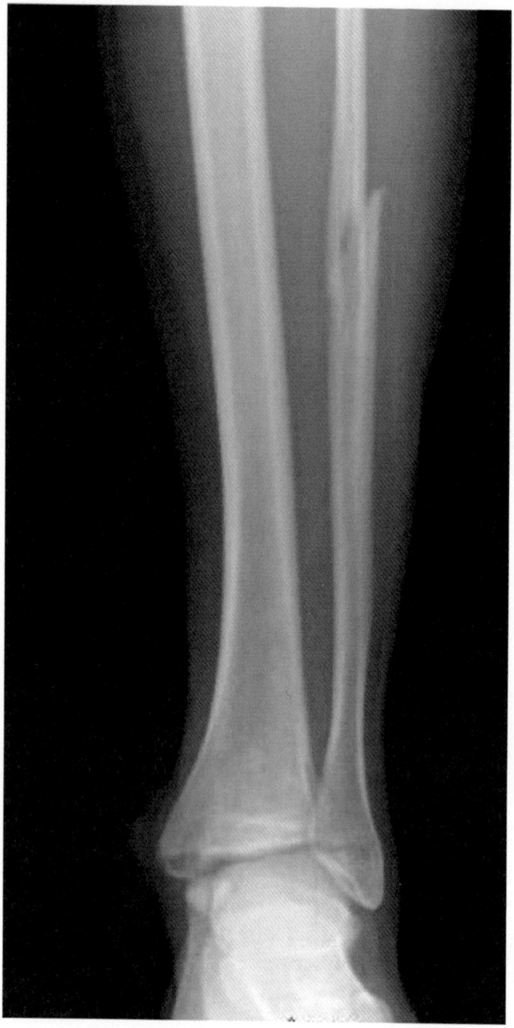

FIGURE 7.3 AP radiograph of the left tibia, revealing an associated proximal fibular shaft fracture

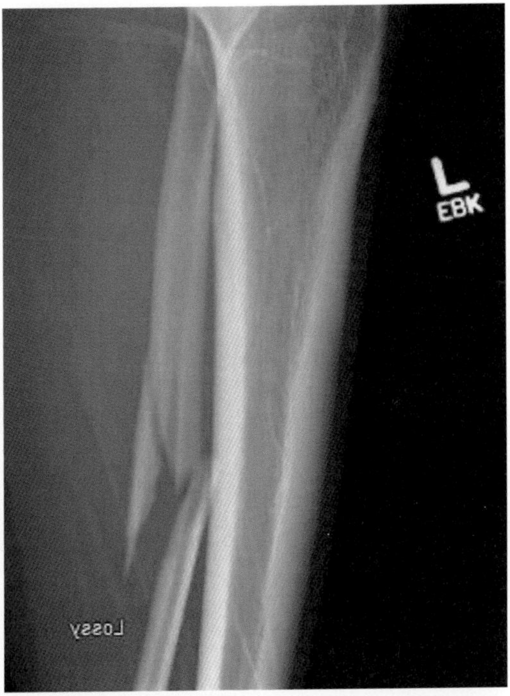

FIGURE 7.4 Lateral radiograph of the left tibia, revealing an associated proximal fibular shaft fracture

Treatment

After the patient was anesthetized and placed supine on the operative table, the leg was sterilely prepped. Contralateral fluoroscopic imaging was obtained as a guide for syndesmotic reduction.

Attention was paid first to the medial malleolus fracture. A standard medial approach was generated, and the medial malleolus was reduced under direct vision. Surgical stabilization was achieved with partially threaded cancellous lag screws (Fig. 7.5). The wound was closed in standard fashion.

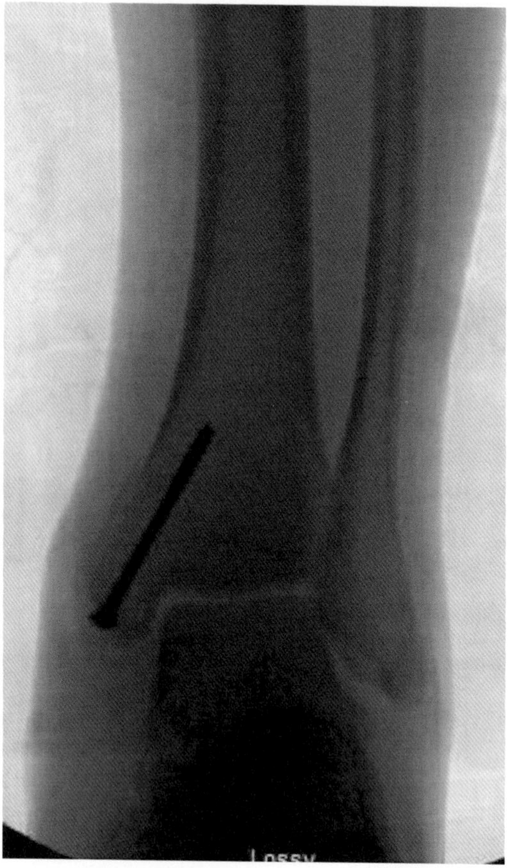

FIGURE 7.5 Intraoperative fluoroscopic image, demonstrating stabilization of the medial malleolus fracture

Next, attention was paid to the fibula. Because the fibula was not significantly shortened and rotated (as compared to the contralateral fluoroscopic imaging), the fibula fracture proximally did not undergo open reduction and internal fixation. A collinear clamp was utilized to help obtain and maintain syndesmotic reduction. Adequacy of syndesmotic reduction was

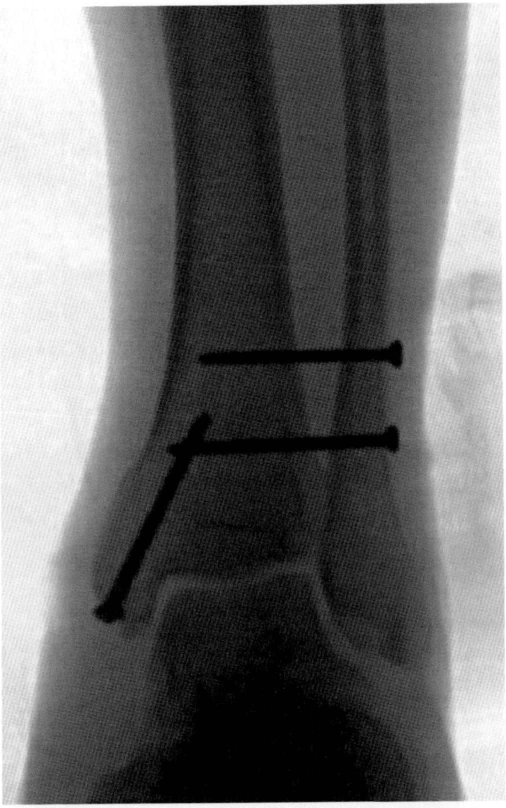

FIGURE 7.6 Intraoperative fluoroscopic image, demonstrating stabilization of the syndesmosis with two 3.5-mm tricortical screws

based on comparisons to the contralateral fluoroscopic imaging, utilizing the position of the fibula along the tibial plafond laterally as the primary gauge for reduction. With the reduction held, two 3.5-mm cortex screws were applied in tricortical fashion (Fig. 7.6). After the clamp was removed, fluoroscopic imaging verified adequacy of implant position, maintenance of acceptable reduction, and mortise stability (with Cotton stress tests). The wound was closed in standard fashion.

Rehabilitation

The patient was kept nonweight bearing for approximately 8 weeks. He was permitted to perform range of motion as tolerated. He was allowed to progress with partial weight bearing after 9–12 weeks. At his 12-week post-op mark, he was permitted to be full weight bearing with a CAM walking boot.

Discussions were held with the patient regarding the risks and benefits of syndesmotic screw removal versus retention, and the patient elected to retain the screws.

At the last follow-up at 9 months, the patient had returned to activities and sports without limitations (Figs. 7.7 and 7.8).

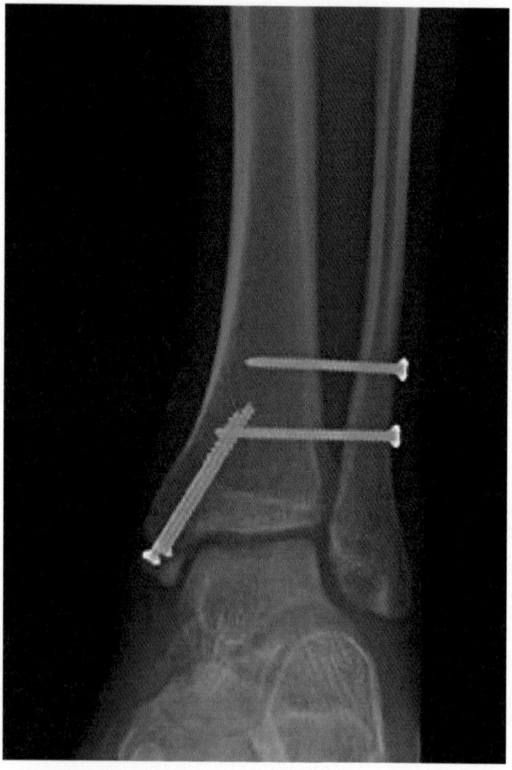

FIGURE 7.7 AP radiograph of the left ankle at the patient's 9-month postoperative mark

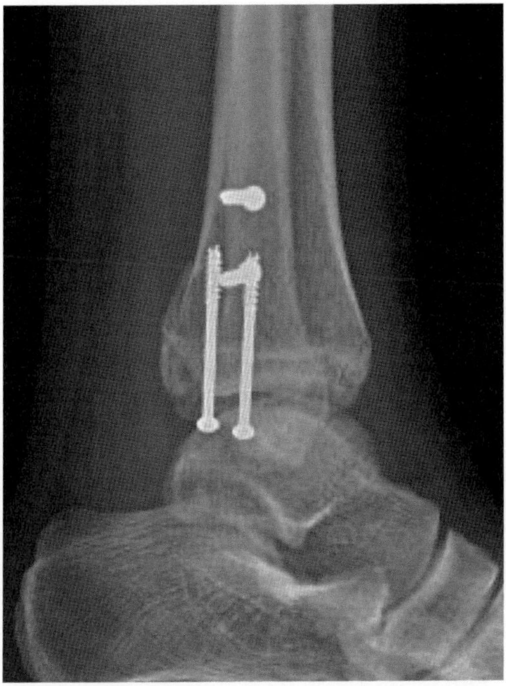

FIGURE 7.8 Lateral radiograph of the left ankle at the patient's 9-month postoperative mark

Salient Points/Pearls

- Maissoneuve fractures are associated with extensive interosseous disruption and syndesmotic instability. Because of the higher position of the fibular fractures, these injuries can be potentially missed on standard ankle radiographic series. Therefore, in addition to obtaining a complete ankle radiographic series, full-length tibia/fibula radiographs are also warranted.
- The absence of fibular and medial malleolus fractures does not rule out the presence of syndesmotic injuries. Such variants include ligamentous deltoid disruptions (which act similarly to a medial malleolus fracture) and/or significant interosseous membrane disruption without a

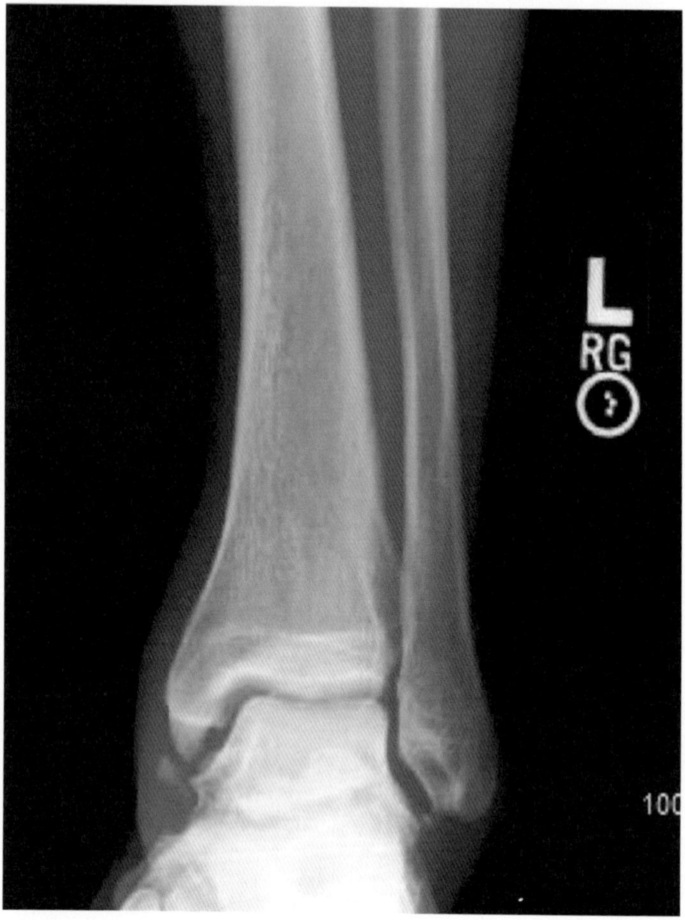

FIGURE 7.9 AP radiograph of a left ankle, revealing a subtle avulsion fracture of the medial malleolus

concomitant fibular fracture (Figs. 7.9 and 7.10). Although these variants are less common, these must be adequately evaluated and excluded.

- Stress radiographs are necessary in order to determine the stability of the ankle joint (Fig. 7.11) and, when coupled with proximal tibia/fibula radiographs, help reveal the diagnosis (Figs. 7.12 and 7.13).

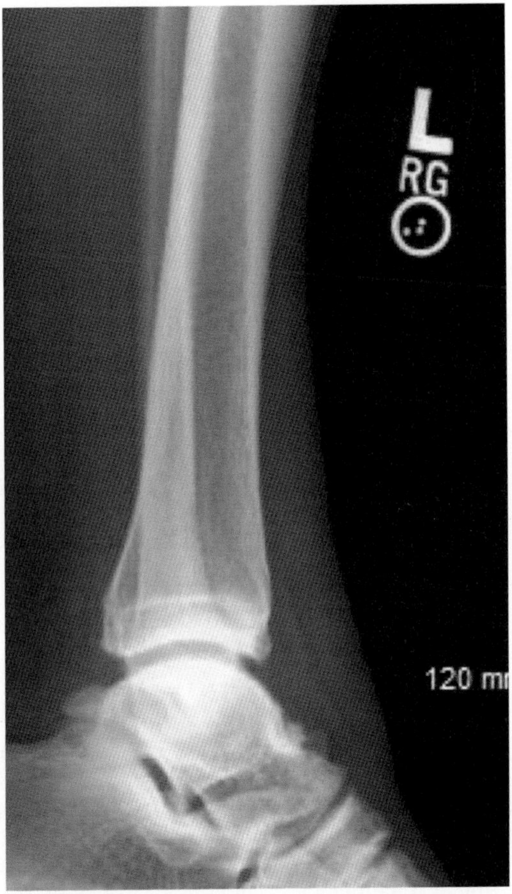

FIGURE 7.10 Lateral radiograph of a left ankle, revealing a subtle avulsion fracture of the medial malleolus

- Additionally, the patient may also respond to provocative tests, such as the squeeze and external rotation stress tests. The squeeze test is performed by applying a compressive force between the fibula and the tibia superior to the mid-point of the calf with the knee bent at 90°. A positive test indicates syndesmotic injury. The external rotation test is positive if pain is reproduced with external rotation of the foot and ankle relative to the tibia. Caution should be used

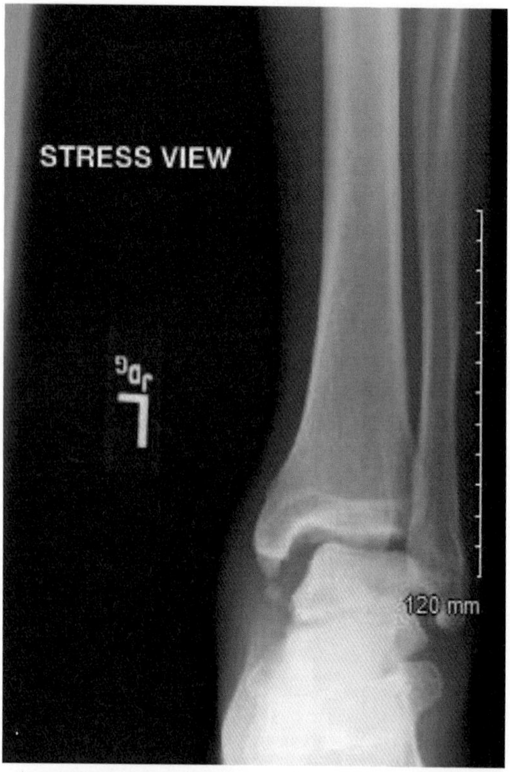

FIGURE 7.11 Stress view of the left ankle (from Figs. 7.9 and 7.10), revealing medial clear space widening. Because of the absence of a "visualized" fibular fracture, the physician must assume the presence of a fibular fracture and/or syndesmotic instability as contributory elements to the patient's ankle instability

to stabilize the tibia but not the fibula during this test to avoid a false-negative result [1].

- Treatment for Maissoneuve fractures requires anatomic reduction of the syndesmosis and stabilization of the ankle mortise; this is accomplished through reduction of the fracture(s) and syndesmosis. Stabilization must be accomplished along the medial column (medial malleolus or

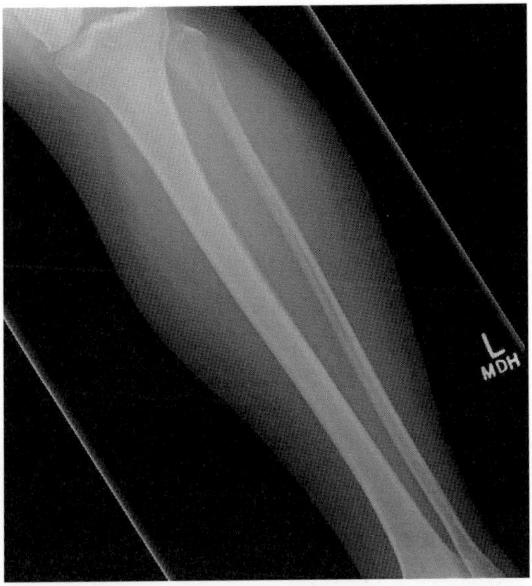

FIGURE 7.12 AP radiograph of the left tibia (from Figs. 7.9 and 7.10), confirming the presence of a proximal fibular fracture

deltoid ligament disruption) and the lateral column (syndesmosis and fibula). To accomplish reduction of the syndesmosis in the setting of a high fibular fracture, open reduction of the fibular fracture to correct length and rotation can result in improved anatomic reduction of the syndesmosis [2]. Stabilization of the syndesmosis can be accomplished with screws of varying configurations or suture techniques, as controversy exists as to the optimal methodology and construct for stabilization.

- Reduction and fixation of the medial malleolus is accomplished through standard techniques. In cases of deltoid ligament disruption, primary repair may be warranted when the mortise does not adequately reduce despite adequacy of fibular reduction. In such instances, suspected interposition of capsular tissues or hematoma may block reduction [3].

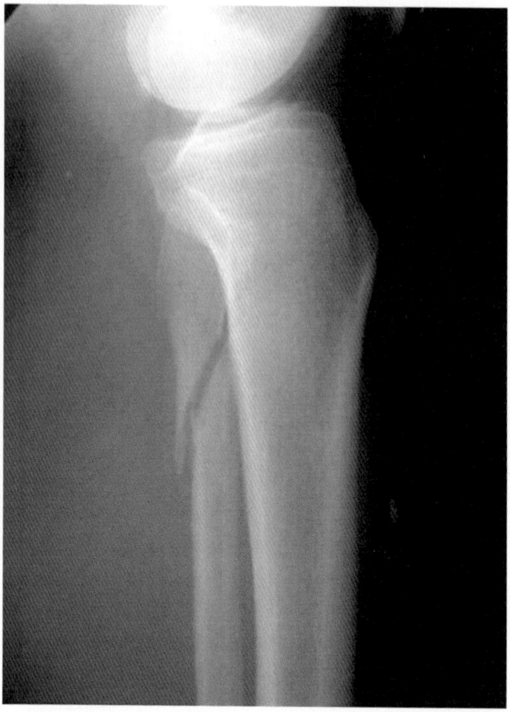

FIGURE 7.13 Lateral radiograph of the left tibia (from Figs. 7.9 and 7.10), confirming the presence of a proximal fibular fracture

- For postoperative rehabilitation, most surgeons recommend a period of nonweight bearing for a minimum of 6 weeks to prevent fixation failure, while others have recommended 12 weeks of nonweight bearing to allow for further ligamentous healing [4]. Furthermore, the role of routine syndesmotic hardware removal also remains controversial [5, 6]. The author does not recommend routine removal of the screws and keeps these patients nonweight bearing for 8 weeks.

References

1. Hunt KJ, Phisitkul P, Pirolo J, Amendola A. High ankle sprains and syndesmotic injuries in athletes. J Am Acad Orthop Surg. 2015;23(11):661–73.
2. Pelton K, Thordarson DB, Barnwell J. Open versus closed treatment of the fibula in Maissoneuve injuries. Foot Ankle Int. 2010;31(7):604–8.
3. Stufkens SA, van den Bekerom MP, Knupp M, Hintermann B, van Dijk CN. The diagnosis and treatment of deltoid ligament lesions in supination-external rotation ankle fractures: a review. Strategies Trauma Limb Reconstr. 2012;7(2):73–8.
4. American Orthopaedic Foot and Ankle Society: Treatment of syndesmosis disruptions. http://www.aofas.org/education/orthopaedicarticles/treatment- of-syndesmosis-disruptions.pdf. Accessed 2 Sep 2015.
5. Schepers T, van Zuuren WJ, van den Bekerom MP, Vogels LM, van Lieshout EM. The management of acute distal tibio-fibular syndesmotic injuries: results of a nationwide survey. Injury. 2012;43(10):1718–23.
6. Hamid N, Loeffler BJ, Braddy W, Kellam JF, Cohen BE, Bosse MJ. Outcome after fixation of ankle fractures with an injury to the syndesmosis: the effect of the syndesmosis screw. J Bone Joint Surg Br. 2009;91(8):1069–73.

Chapter 8
Maisonneuve Fractures: Syndesmotic Fixation Using Plate

Natalie R. Danna and Nirmal C. Tejwani

Case Presentation

The patient is a 25-year-old male who presents with right ankle and leg pain after an assault. He reports that his leg was twisted and stomped on by the perpetrators. He had immediate pain and inability to weight bear.

Examination revealed diffuse swelling over the ankle. He was tender to palpation over the lateral malleolus and proximal fibula. He was also tender over the posterior malleolus but not over the remainder of the tibia.

Injury Films

Full-length films of the tibia (AP and lateral) and ankle (AP, lateral, mortise) were obtained. They demonstrated an

---

N.R. Danna, M.D. • N.C. Tejwani, M.D. (✉)
Department of Orthopedics, NYU Langone Medical Center, New York, NY, USA
e-mail: nirmal.tejwani@nyumc.org

N.C. Tejwani (ed.), *Fractures of the Foot and Ankle*,
DOI 10.1007/978-3-319-60456-5_8,

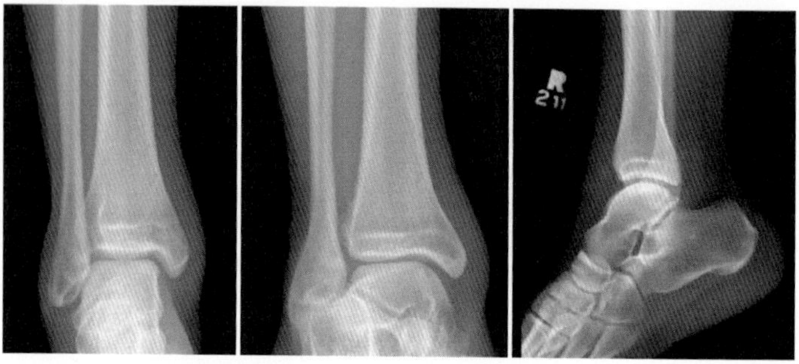

FIGURE 8.1 AP, mortise, and lateral radiographs of the injury

oblique fracture of the proximal fibula and widening of the ankle mortise (Fig. 8.1).

Diagnostic Testing and Treatment Considerations

Medial clear space widening greater than 5 mm indicates a tear of the deltoid ligament with accompanying disruption of the distal tibiofibular syndesmosis, which should be surgically stabilized. An external rotation stress radiograph was performed to assess syndesmotic integrity, and frank widening of the ankle mortise was observed (Fig. 8.2).

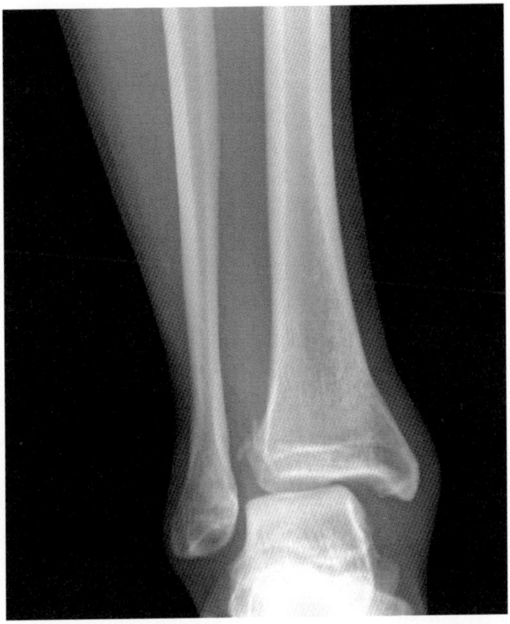

FIGURE 8.2 External rotation stress view demonstrates widening of the syndesmosis and medial clear space

Treatment and Timing of Surgery

At initial evaluation, the patient was placed into a well-padded, short-leg AO splint, with radiographic confirmation of reduction of the ankle mortise. He was instructed to remain nonweightbearing on that extremity and maintain elevation of the limb as much as possible. Surgery was scheduled few days after injury (7 days) to allow decrease of swelling and improvement of the condition of the soft tissues.

Surgical Tact

Surgical intervention for Maisonneuve injuries is focused on reduction and fixation of the syndesmosis [1, 2]. This is generally accomplished with one or two 3.5 mm tri- or quadri-cortical screws. The distal screw should be placed approximately 2 cm proximal to the plafond, and the second screw should be placed 1–2 cm proximal to that. While there is debate in the literature about the number and size of screws as well as whether they should extend to the fourth cortex [3], the authors prefer a minimum of two screws of 3.5 mm diameter (tri- or quadri-cortical) for these syndesmotic injuries.

A short plate may be used to disperse the forces exerted by the screws and help with centralizing the screws on the fibula.

The proximal shaft fibula fracture does not generally require fixation unless significantly shortened and hindering syndesmosis reduction [1, 2, 4]. If needed, a small incision may be made over the fibula fracture site and length regained using a clamp before syndesmosis fixation.

Technique of Open Reduction and Internal Fixation

To accommodate the plate, an incision of approximately 3 cm was made over the fibula, and a lateral approach was made. The three-hole one-third tubular plate was centered on the fibula, and the foot was dorsiflexed. Using a large pointed reduction clamp with one tine on the fibula through the middle hole of the plate and the other tine medially on the tibia, the syndesmosis was reduced. This reduction was confirmed radiographically, as seen by normal medial and syndesmosis clear spaces. All four cortices were drilled with a 2.5 mm drill, and two tricortical 3.5 mm screws were placed (Fig. 8.3).

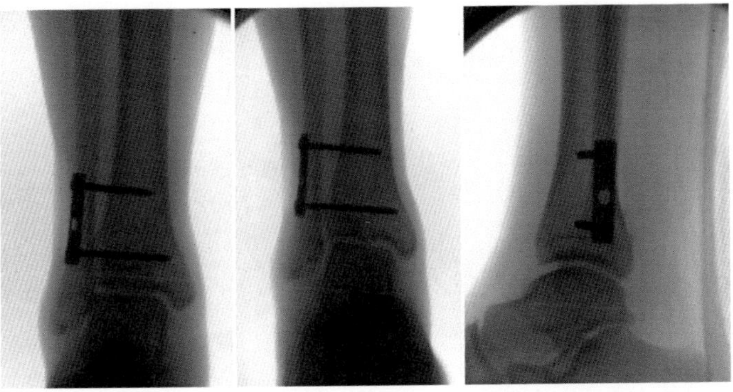

FIGURE 8.3 AP, mortise, and lateral intraoperative radiographs demonstrating fixation

Fluoroscopy was used to confirm reduction of the syndesmosis, as well as the proximal fibula fracture. It is important to check that the fibula length has been regained; on the mortise view, the "dime" sign is useful [4].

The patient was placed in a short leg splint for 2 weeks after surgery.

Postoperative Plan

The splint was removed at 2 weeks and replaced with a cam boot, with instructions for the patient to start ankle range of motion exercises. Follow-up X-rays are shown in Fig. 8.4. The patient was kept nonweightbearing for a period of 12 weeks.

After this period, he was also referred to physical therapy. The patient was informed of the risk of screw breakage, but we do not perform routine removal of tricortical screws, though the patient is informed of the likelihood of screw loosening or breakage as will be noted on the follow-up radiographs.

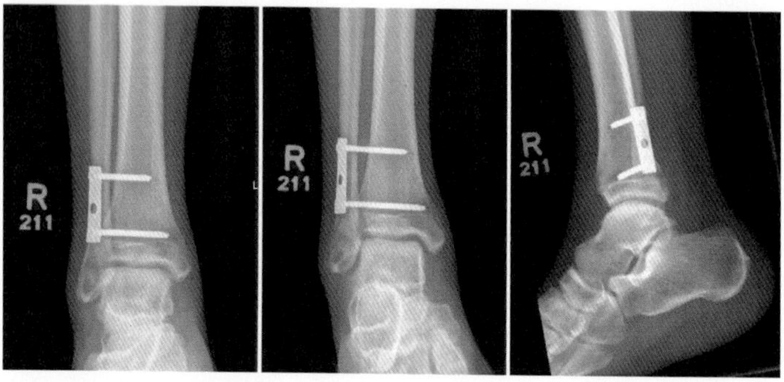

FIGURE 8.4 AP, mortise, and lateral radiographs at follow-up visit

Outcomes

Lambers et al. reported on radiographic and functional outcomes after operative fixation of syndesmotic injuries [5]. At an average of 21 years postoperatively, 49% of patients had “substantial” radiographic arthritis [5]. However, the radiographic findings were not a significant predictor of functional outcome: 92% of patients in the series had good or excellent AOFAS scores. The authors found that patient-reported pain was the most significant predictor of outcome at follow-up [5].

At an average of 6 years postoperatively, Babis et al. found ankle range of motion equivalent to the contralateral side in 79% of their patients [6].

Studies of the syndesmosis after operative fixation by Gennis et al. have shown that there is only mild widening (less than 0.5 mm) of the tibiofibular clear space after initiation of weightbearing [7]. The ankle mortise remains congruent, however, whether the syndesmotic screws remain intact, break, or are removed [7].

Salient Points/Pearls

- Goal of treatment: congruent and reduced ankle mortise and syndesmosis.
- High fibula fracture rarely requires internal fixation.

- Syndesmotic screws may engage 3 or 4 cortices and may be 1 or 2 in number.
- Patients should remain nonweightbearing for 6–12 weeks after internal fixation based on injury pattern, patient size, and fixation used. (The author prefers two screws if only syndesmosis fixation done.)
- Return of near normal pre-injury function is expected, despite radiographic evidence of posttraumatic arthritis.

References

1. Duchesneau S, Fallat LM. The Maisonneuve fracture. J Foot Ankle Surg. 1995;34(5):422–8.
2. Kalyani BS, Roberts CS, Giannoudis PV. The Maisonneuve injury: a comprehensive review. Orthopedics. 2010;33(3):196–7.
3. Wikerøy AK, Høiness PR, Andreassen GS, Hellund JC, Madsen JE. No difference in functional and radiographic results 8.4 years after quadricortical compared with tricortical syndesmosis fixation in ankle fractures. J Orthop Trauma. 2010;24(1):17–23.
4. White TO, Bugler KE. Ankle fractures. In: Court-Brown C, Heckman JD, et al., editors. Rockwood and Green's: fractures in adults. 8th ed. Philadelphia: Orthopaedic Publications; 2015. p. 2542–86.
5. Lambers KT, van den Bekerom MP, Doornberg JN, Stufkens SA, van Dijk CN, Kloen P. Long-term outcome of pronation-external rotation ankle fractures treated with syndesmotic screws only. J Bone Joint Surg Am. 2013;95(17):e1221–7.
6. Babis GC, Papagelopoulos PJ, Tsarouchas J, Zoubos AB, Korres DS, Nikiforidis P. Operative treatment for Maisonneuve fracture of the proximal fibula. Orthopedics. 2000;23(7):687–90.
7. Gennis E, Koenig S, Rodericks D, Otlans P, Tornetta P 3rd. The fate of the fixed syndesmosis over time. Foot Ankle Int. 2015;36(10):1202–8.

Chapter 9
Calcaneus Fracture: Extended Lateral Approach

Neil Sardesai, Mark Gage, and Marcus Sciadini

Case

The patient is a 44-year-old male who sustained a closed injury to his left hindfoot after a fall from height.

On physical examination, his left hindfoot was grossly swollen, ecchymotic, with notable heel widening. He was diffusely tender to palpation along the medial and lateral aspects of his heel. No neurovascular deficits were noted. Radiographs (Fig. 9.1a, b) demonstrate a right calcaneus fracture with intra-articular extension into the posterior facet.

The left lower extremity was immobilized in a bulky cotton short-leg splint with strict elevation precautions to assist with edema control. A CT scan was obtained to further evaluate the injury. This revealed two displaced fracture lines

N. Sardesai, M.D. • M. Gage, M.D. • M. Sciadini, M.D. (✉)
Department of Orthopaedics, University of Maryland School of Medicine, R. Adams Cowley Shock Trauma Center, Baltimore, MD, USA
e-mail: msciadini@umoa.umm.edu

N.C. Tejwani (ed.), *Fractures of the Foot and Ankle*,
DOI 10.1007/978-3-319-60456-5_9,

extending into the posterior facet (Sanders type 3 AC [1, 2]) with lateral wall diastasis and calcaneal tuberosity varus angulation (Fig. 9.2a–c).

The patient was indicated for surgical treatment and underwent open reduction and internal fixation using an extended lateral approach. Postoperatively, the patient remained non-weightbearing for a total of 8 weeks. Sutures were removed at 2 weeks during which time the patient was transitioned from a splint to a walking boot to allow early ankle and subtalar range of motion.

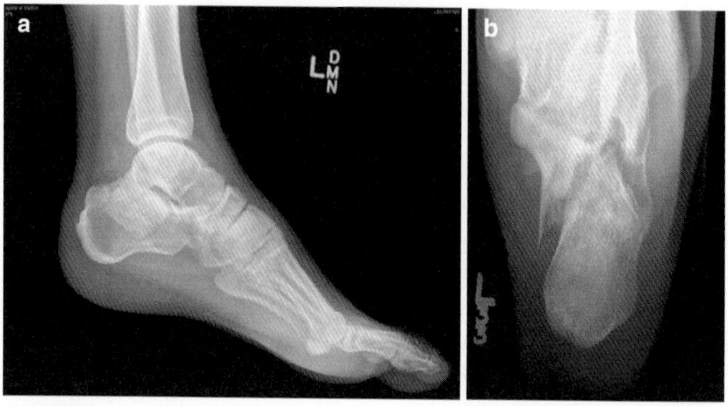

FIGURE 9.1 Injury lateral (**a**) and Harris heel (**b**) views of the hindfoot

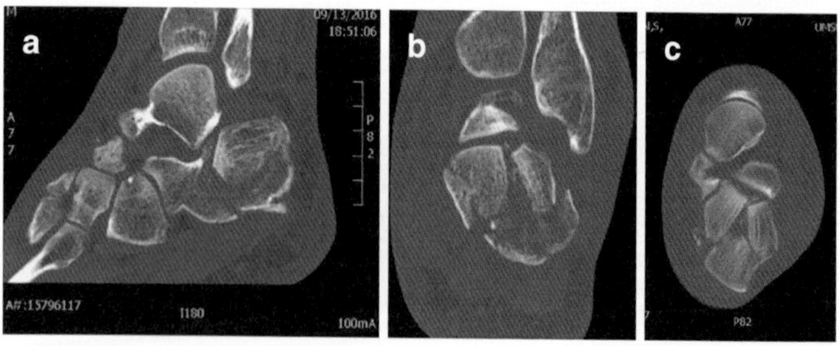

FIGURE 9.2 CT scan images including illustrative sagittal (**a**), coronal (**b**), and axial (**c**) reconstructions

Background

The calcaneus is the most commonly fractured tarsal bone and can be very challenging to treat. Injury is usually the result of direct axial loading to the heel most commonly due to falls from height or motor vehicle collisions. Spine fractures or contralateral calcaneus fractures can occur in 10–15% of patients. Functionally, the calcaneus is important in support of the entirety of body weight with ambulation, hindfoot range of motion through the subtalar joint, and appropriate force transmission from the hindfoot to the midfoot during normal gait.

Imaging

Obtaining appropriate imaging is essential to characterizing the fracture pattern and developing a plan for reduction and fixation. Basic imaging should include AP, lateral, and Harris axial heel view radiographs as well as computed tomography (CT scans). One should evaluate the obtained imaging for the following characteristics: posterior facet joint depression, coronal malalignment and diastasis, the extent of calcaneal tuberosity shortening and angulation as well as the presence and extent of intra-articular involvement. Intraoperatively, contralateral lateral and Harris view fluoroscopic images are helpful for comparative purposes when assessing reduction.

Indications

All displaced calcaneus fractures are amenable to open reduction and internal fixation. Contraindications to surgical treatment may include smokers who are unwilling to abstain from smoking, vasculopathic patients, uncontrolled diabetic patients, and elderly, low-demand patients. Nondisplaced or minimally displaced fractures may also be managed nonoperatively [3].

Relative indications for surgery include poor heel position and shape, displaced articular involvement, no medical contraindications to operative care, open fractures, compliant patients younger than 60 years of age, and nonsmokers [4].

Surgical fixation aims to reduce the fractured calcaneus to its normal anatomy, restore the critical angle of Gissane as well as Bohler's angle, and recreate the congruity of the subtalar joint [3]. Anatomic reduction of the articular surface and correction of the typical deformities affecting the tuberosity (varus angulation, shortening, flattening, and widening) are the surgical goals with the goal of minimizing the long-term risk of symptomatic subtalar arthritis and facilitating normal shoe wear and hindfoot mechanics [5]. Rigid internal fixation allows for early motion of the ankle and subtalar joints.

Soft Tissue Management

Most calcaneal fractures are associated with significant soft tissue injury often the result of high energy trauma. In addition to the osseous injury, the soft tissues are significantly affected resulting in a tender, ecchymotic, swollen, and deformed heel [5]. Oftentimes fracture blisters will develop around the hindfoot. Some authors suggest leaving these closed for as long as possible. Our approach is to unroof the blisters early and begin dressing changes to facilitate epithelial repair and potentially shorten the time course to definitive surgery. If still present at the time of definitive fixation, blisters should be unroofed prior to surgical prep to minimize risk of inoculating the surgical wound with bacterial species which frequently colonize the blister fluid.

Vascular Supply

The blood supply to the calcaneus and its overlying soft tissue may predispose it to avascular necrosis and wound healing complications. The calcaneus receives its blood supply from medial and lateral calcaneal arteries [6].

Disruption of the lateral blood supply may result from both the inciting trauma or possibly in during the surgery. Interruption of this blood supply may cause a significant nutrient deficiency in the lateral half of the calcaneus. The remaining blood supply therefore is reliant on the medial penetrating vascularization [6].

Approach

Setup

The patient should be placed in a lateral decubitus position with the operative calcaneus up. Our preference is to use a radiolucent extension to the end of a standard operating room table to allow for more extensive fluoroscopic access. The patient should be brought to the end of the bed so that the foot can be accessed from both sides as well as the end of the Table. A nonsterile tourniquet should be placed above the knee on the operative extremity. The fluoroscopic imager should be positioned orthogonally to the axis of the body. Folded blankets are stacked around and on top of the nonoperative extremity as depicted (Fig. 9.3) to create a flat surface on which to operate.

Landmarks and Incision

After the leg has been prepped and draped, the extensile lateral approach is marked on the skin. The inferior limb of the incision is made performed just anterior to the lateral edge of the Achilles tendon to best preserve the lateral calcaneal artery which is responsible for the majority of the supply to the corner of the soft tissue flap. The inferior limb of the incision is carried at the transition point of the glabrous skin and is carried to the base of the fifth metatarsal. Once the skin and subcutaneous tissue is incised, the soft tissue envelope is sharply elevated as a full-thickness flap including

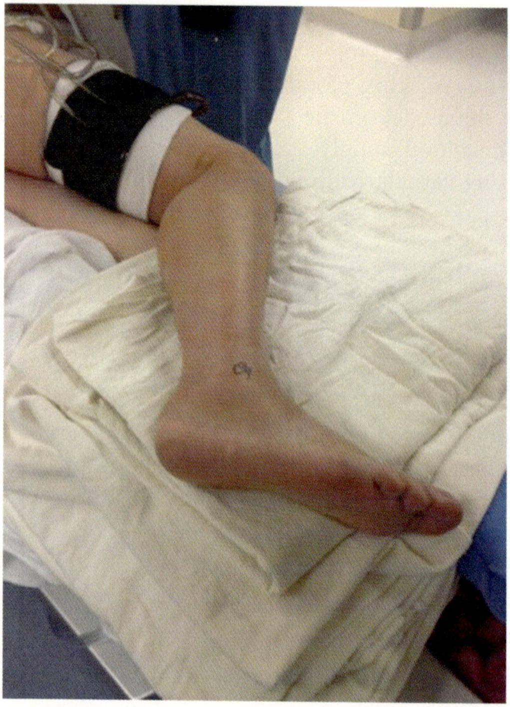

FIGURE 9.3 Lateral positioning of patient on regular OR table demonstrating use of blankets to support lower extremity and provide flat operating surface

release of the calcaneofibular ligament (Fig. 9.4). This is critical to preserving the flap's viability and maximizing surgical site healing. The flap is elevated in a subperiosteal fashion proximally to the subtalar joint and anteriorly to expose the calcaneocuboid joint. The peroneal tendons are also elevated from the peroneal tubercle and reflected dorsally to maximize exposure of the lateral calcaneus and subtalar joint. Kirschner wires are placed into the distal fibula, cuboid, talus, and cuneiforms to serve as retractors and minimize the risk of excessive retraction of the lateral heel flap. Grasping of the skin edges with forceps or use of self-retaining retractors

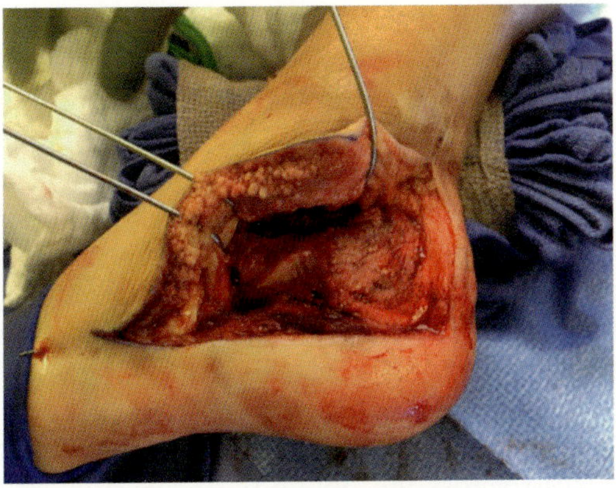

FIGURE 9.4 Intraoperative clinical photo showing full-thickness soft tissue flap elevated and K-wires providing retraction

should be minimized during flap elevation and skin hooks are a preferred mode of retraction to minimize surgical trauma to the soft tissues.

Caution

The lateral extensile approach to the calcaneus has been associated with a high soft tissue complication and infection rate, in some instances as high as 25% [1, 3].

Reduction Maneuver

The use of the lateral approach allows excellent exposure to the entire calcaneus. This case illustrates a classic fracture pattern where the posterior facet articular surface is fractured into multiple segments and depressed plantarly. The calcaneal tuberosity becomes angulated into a hindfoot varus position. The lateral wall of the tuberosity is typically displaced laterally and mobilized during the operation to allow access to the articular fragments (Fig. 9.5). Sequence of surgery varies depending upon surgeon preference, fracture pattern, and displacement. Although the medial portion of the posterior facet articular surface is often assumed to remain in a reduced position, elevation of this fragment against the inferior surface of the talus is often necessary to provide a stable reference for reduction of the impacted lateral articular fragments. These lateral fragments may need to be temporarily mobilized further laterally while the tuberosity reduction is performed since shortening of the tuberosity may block the ability to elevate the lateral articular fragments into an anatomically reduced position. An osteotome can be placed across the obliquity of this primary fracture line beneath the posterior facet and used to lever the calcaneal tuberosity out of varus angulation, bring the tuberosity out to appropriate length, and restore height. This maneuver may be aided by placement of a 5.0 mm Schanz pin into the tuberosity (Figs. 9.6 and 9.7). A separate V-shaped cortical fragment defining the angle of Gissane is often present between the posterior facet and anterior process and reduction of this fragment often facilitates restoration of the

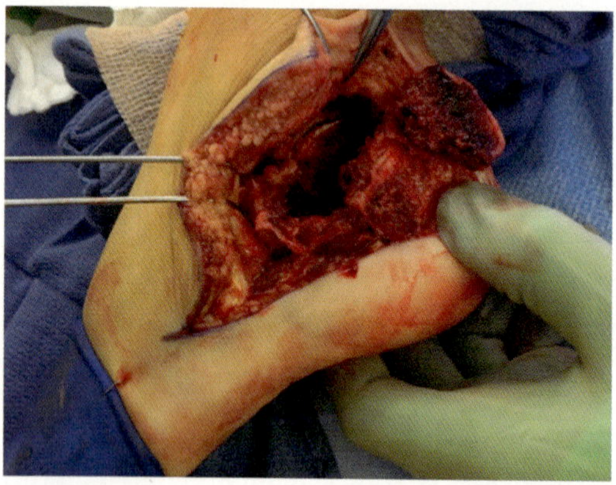

Figure 9.5 Intraoperative clinical photo showing mobilization of lateral wall fragment to reveal intra-articular impaction of the lateral articular surface of the subtalar joint and medial articular "constant fragment"

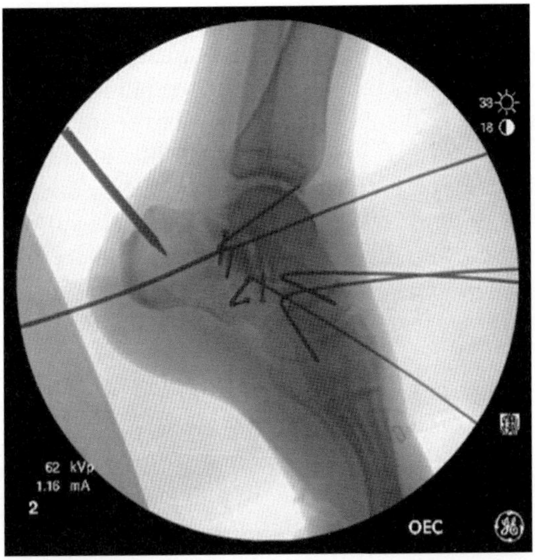

FIGURE 9.6 Intraoperative lateral fluoroscopic image demonstrating reduction of articular surface with mini-fragment lag-screw fixation and restoration of calcaneal tuberosity height and length

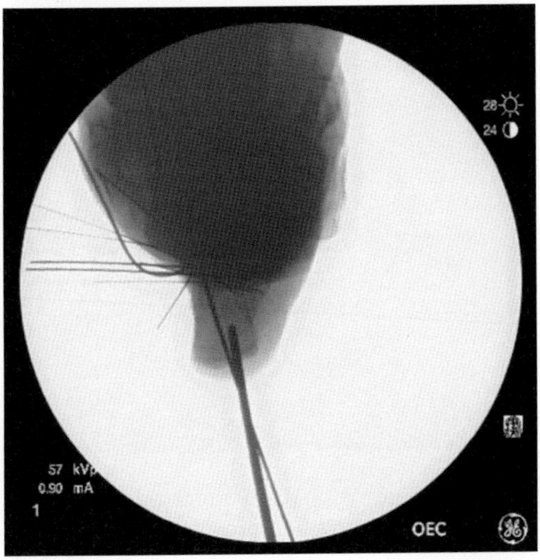

FIGURE 9.7 Intraoperative Harris heel fluoroscopic image demonstrating correction of varus malalignment of calcaneal tuberosity

relationship between these structures and may precede or follow elevation of and anatomic reduction of the depressed lateral articular fragments. Multiple small-diameter smooth K-wires provide provisional fixation of the multiple reduced fracture fragments (Figs. 9.6 and 9.8) while lateral and Harris heel fluoroscopic imaging confirms the reduction. Once reduction is confirmed, wires can be replaced with mini-fragment screws and a laterally based plate to buttress the lateral cortex and provide fixed-angle raft screw support of the articular surface (Fig. 9.9).

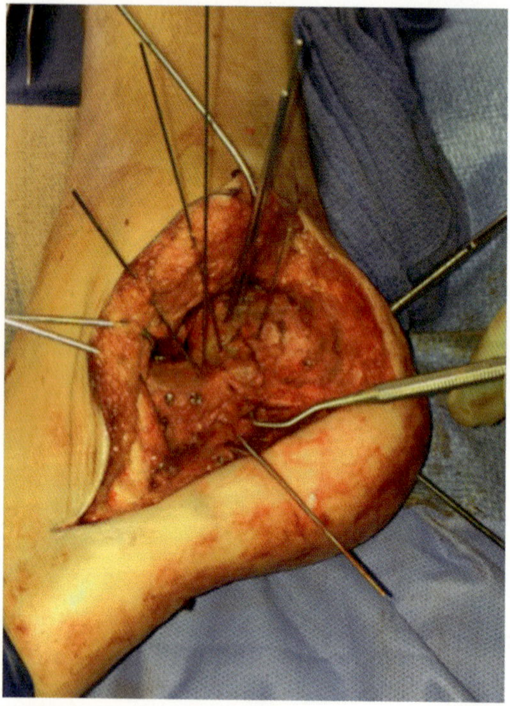

FIGURE 9.8 Intraoperative photo demonstrating reduced fracture with mini-fragment lag-screw and provisional K-wire fixation

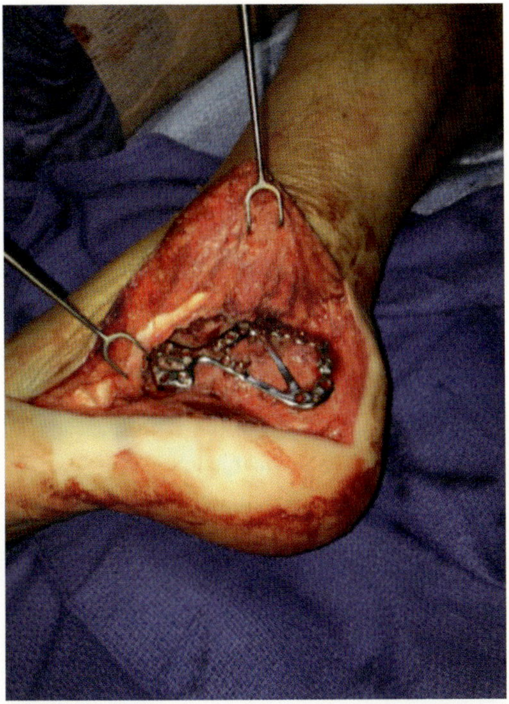

FIGURE 9.9 Final fixation construct consisting of precontoured locking calcaneal plate

Closure

Closure consists of interrupted 3-0 vicryl sutures in the dermis. Placement of all dermal sutures prior to knot-tying has been advocated, but we prefer to tie each knot as the suture is placed. We do recommend starting closure at the corner and working outward (distally and proximally) to avoid translating skin edges inadvertently. To minimize surgical trauma to the flap, the skin is then reapproximated with 3-0 nylon sutures applied in an Allgower-Donati fashion (Fig. 9.10). Final fluoroscopic images confirm the reduction (Fig. 9.11a, b).

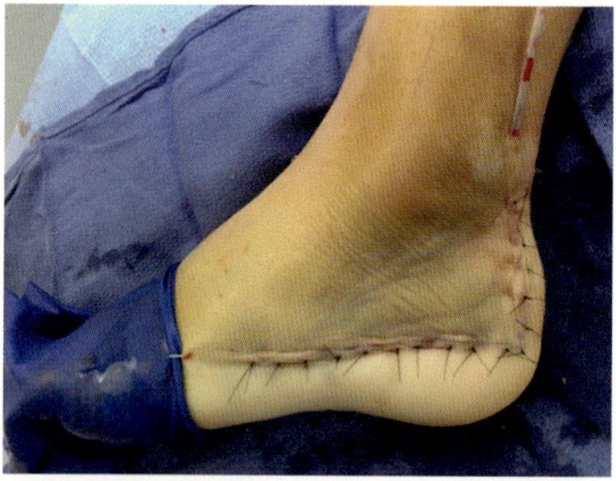

Figure 9.10 Final wound closure over drain with 3-0 nylon sutures placed using Allgower-Donati technique

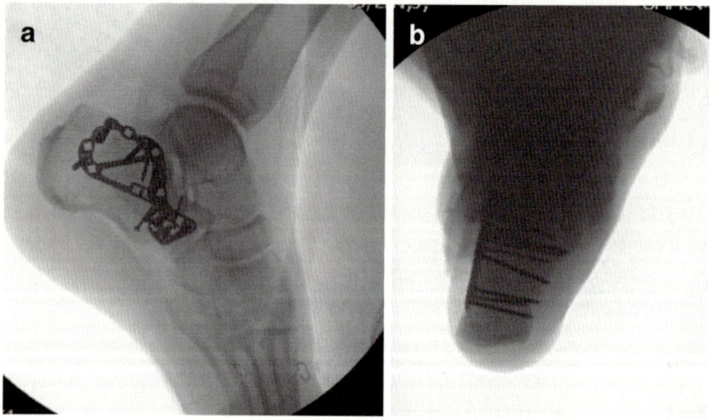

Figure 9.11 Final postoperative lateral (**a**) and Harris heel (**b**) fluoroscopic views

Salient Points/Pearls

- Hindfoot varus can be difficult to correct since the surgical approach is laterally based. A 5.0 mm Schanz pin placed in the postero-superior aspect of the calcaneal tuberosity allows for multiplanar manipulation of this fragment to assist in restoration of length, height, and valgus alignment.
- Kirschner wires allow for maintenance of provisional reduction. These wires may be applied lateral to medial or may be placed percutaneously from the tuberosity into the posterior facet to maintain proper height.
- A lamina spreader can be a useful tool to restore tuberosity length and height and posterior facet height during surgical reduction.
- Bone grafting is rarely indicated in calcaneus surgery. Although large cancellous bone voids may frequently be present between the posterior facet and posterior tuberosity secondary to comminution or impaction, these usually heal uneventfully without grafting in the calcaneus. When necessary, cancellous allograft chips may be used.
- Bone graft substitutes are usually not necessary nor worth the additional cost. Tri-cortical allograft may also be used to augment the axial stability in rare cases.

References

1. Bruce J. Surgical versus conservative interventions for displaced intra-articular calcaneal fractures. Cochrane Database Syst Rev. 2012;1:CD008628. doi:10.1002/14651858.
2. Zuckerman JD, Koval KJ. Handbook of fractures (book). J Bone Joint Surg Am. 2002;84-A(12):2324.
3. Buckley R, Tough S, McCormack R, et al. Operative compared with nonoperative treatment of displaced intra-articular calcaneal fractures: a prospective, randomized, controlled multicenter trial. J Bone Joint Surg Am. 2002;84-A(10):1733–44.
4. Howard JL, Buckley R, McCormack R, et al. Complications following management of displaced intra-articular calcaneal frac-

tures: a prospective randomized trial comparing open reduction internal fixation with nonoperative management. J Orthop Trauma. 2003;17(4):241–9.
5. Sanders R. Displaced intra-articular fractures of the calcaneus. J Bone Joint Surg Am. 2000;82(2):225–50.
6. Andermahr J, Helling HJ, Rehm KE, Koebke Z. The vascularization of the os calcaneum and the clinical consequences. Clin Orthop. 1999;363:212–8.

Chapter 10
Operative Treatment of Calcaneus Fractures Through a Sinus Tarsi Approach

Abhishek Ganta and Philipp Leucht

Case Presentation

A 19-year-old male, intoxicated on LSD, with no significant past medical history was found after a fall from a fire escape. He was brought to the trauma bay by ambulance with bilateral upper and lower extremity pain as well as facial pain. His neurovascular exam was intact (motor and sensation) in all extremities. Orthopedic injuries included a left open olecranon fracture, right radial styloid fracture, bilateral patella fractures, and left calcaneus fracture. Radiographs of the calcaneus showed significant joint depression and impaction of the posterior facet.

Injury Films

Lateral radiographs of the heel demonstrated a joint depression type calcaneus fracture with significant flattening of Böhler's angle to 9°. A Harris heel view revealed mild varus

A. Ganta, M.D. • P. Leucht, M.D. (✉)
Department of Orthopaedic Surgery, Hospital for Joint Diseases, New York University School of Medicine, New York, NY, USA
e-mail: philipp.leucht@nyumc.org

N.C. Tejwani (ed.), *Fractures of the Foot and Ankle*,
DOI 10.1007/978-3-319-60456-5_10,

deformity of the tuberosity fragment and heel widening. CT scans in the sagittal and 30-degree semi-coronal plane further delineated the posterior facet involvement with lateral wall blow-out, depression of the lateral aspect of the posterior facet, and intra-articular split in the sagittal plane, indicating a Sanders 3AB fracture (Fig. 10.1a–d).

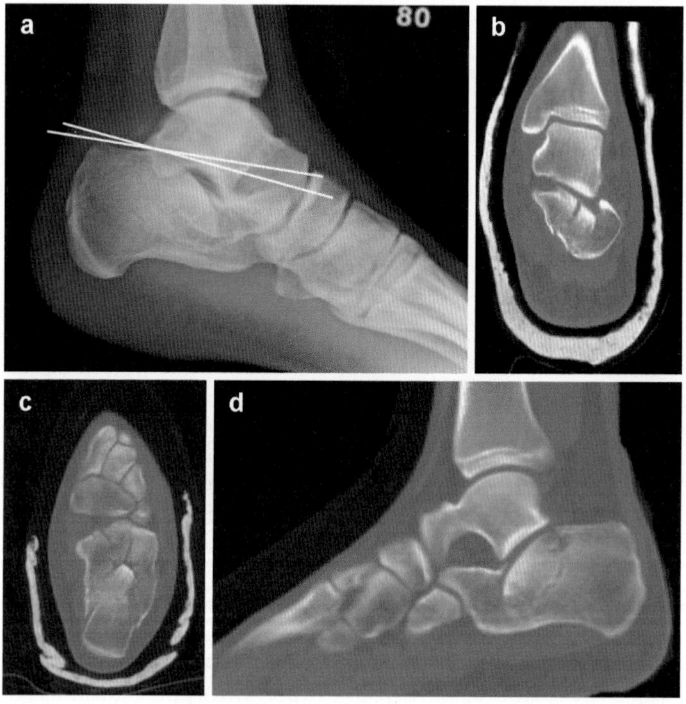

Figure 10.1 Lateral radiograph (**a**), 30-degree semi-coronal (**b**), sagittal (**c**), and axial (**d**) CT showing an intra-articular joint depression type calcaneus fracture. There is flattening of the Böhler's angle to 9° and joint depression with impaction on the lateral radiograph (**a**). The 30-degree semi-coronal plane view (**b**) allows for the Sander's Classification as well as further defining the involvement of the posterior facet. The axial CT cut shows medial cortex overlap indicating varus alignment of the calcaneus (**c**). The sagittal cut demonstrates posterior facet depression (**d**)

Treatment and Timing of Surgery

The decision was made together with the patient to address his calcaneus fracture with open reduction internal fixation in an attempt to restore articular congruency and thus decrease the potential risk for post-traumatic arthritis of the subtalar joint. Historically, patients with similar calcaneus fractures were instructed to elevate their injured extremity for up to 3 weeks until soft tissue swelling had subsided and an extensile L-shaped approach could be performed safely without risking postoperative wound complications. Complication rates with the extensile approach reached from 1.5% in experienced hands to 30% in the general literature [1].

Recently, the limited incision sinus tarsi approach has gained traction and is now commonly used at our institution for the treatment of calcaneus fractures. Due to the shorter incision, and more proximal location of the incision, wound complications are less common [2]. However, because of the smaller surgical window, visualization is more difficult, often relying on indirect reduction techniques [3]. These indirect reduction maneuvers are easily performed within the first 7–10 days, after which fracture fragments become "sticky" and anatomic reduction is often more difficult to obtain [4]. In this case scenario, the soft tissue swelling was minimal and there was no blistering; therefore the patient was taken to the operating room on day seven after his injury.

Surgical Tact

Position

Lateral decubitus position with a beanbag on a radiolucent operating room table with the foot at the very distal aspect of the table. The operative leg is positioned on a bone foam positioner. Alternatively, a towel ramp can be built, creating a flat surface to rest the operative leg. The fluoroscopy unit is brought in obliquely from the contralateral side (Fig. 10.2a). A thigh tourniquet is placed.

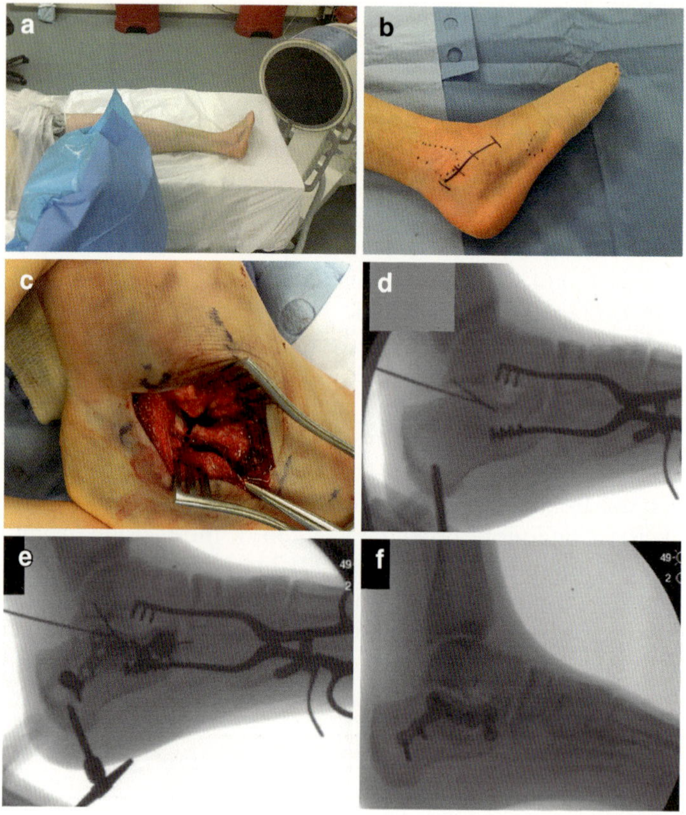

FIGURE 10.2 Intraoperative setup demonstrates lateral decubitus positioning with the operative leg on a radiolucent bone foam positioner (**a**). Note that this allows for the fluoroscopy unit to be brought in from the contralateral side to help obtain a Harris heel view. A 4–6 cm incision is made over the sinus tarsi (**b**) using the inferior aspect of the fibula and the fourth metatarsal base as bony landmarks. Intraoperative image (**c**) and fluoroscopy (**d**) show the use of a periosteal elevator underneath the posterior facet to achieve reduction along with the use of a percutaneous Schanz pin in the tuberosity to reduce the varus deformity. Further intraoperative fluoroscopic views showing plate placement on the lateral aspect of the calcaneus 5 mm distal to the posterior facet joint line (**e**, **f**)

Approach

After exsanguination of the limb, a 4–6 cm incision is made over the sinus tarsi (Fig. 10.2b). Bony landmarks include the inferior aspect of the fibula and the fourth metatarsal base. If swelling or body habitus precludes palpation of bony prominence, a K-wire may be placed on the skin coursing from the inferior aspect of the fibula in line with the fourth metatarsal and position can be verified with fluoroscopy. Careful soft tissue dissection is carried down to the peroneal tendons and extensor digitorum brevis; very rarely will branches of the sural nerve come into the field [5–7]. The retinaculum over the peroneal tendons is incised and the tendons are retracted carefully out of the field, keeping the tendon sheath intact. The fascia and muscle of the extensor digitorum brevis are also incised and elevated distally. This allows access to the capsular structures, which are subsequently excised to visualize the articular surface of the posterior facet and the angle of Gissane.

Fracture Reduction Techniques and Fixation

After exposure of the subtalar joint, the amount of fracture comminution and lateral wall involvement was appreciated. Because the approach does not allow exposure of the tuberosity, a Steinmann pin was percutaneously placed into the posterior tuberosity and used to distract and reduce the tuberosity out of varus and restore length [5–7].

A number of reduction techniques can be performed to restore the articular surface of the posterior facet; in this case, a periosteal elevator was placed underneath the posterior facet and the facet fragment was elevated together with its subchondral bone and attached cancellous bone (Fig. 10.2c, d). Once anatomic reduction of the posterior facet was achieved and confirmed radiographically, provisional fixation was maintained with K-wires.

After posterior facet and tuberosity reduction, a large bone void was noted underneath the posterior facet. Tricalcium phosphate cement was injected into the void, followed by closure of the lateral wall fragment.

A sinus tarsi plate with percutaneous jig was then placed on the lateral aspect of the calcaneus about 5 mm distal to the posterior facet joint line (Fig. 10.2e, f). Cortical lag screws by technique were used to compress the posterior facet fracture, followed by placement of cortical screws into the tuberosity and anterior process. In this young patient with good bone quality, cortical screws were sufficient to maintain reduction; however, in elderly patients or patients with severe comminution, locking screws may be utilized to achieve adequate fixation [8].

After reduction is confirmed on biplanar fluoroscopy, the tourniquet was deflated and meticulous hemostasis was obtained and the wound was copiously irrigated prior to closure. Placement of a drain is usually not necessary.

Postoperative Plan

A short leg plaster splint was placed and the patient was instructed to be non-weight bearing on the left lower extremity. Antibiotics were given for a total of 24 h postoperatively. Low molecular weight heparin was continued in the perioperative period for 4 weeks.

The patient was made non-weight bearing for a total of 6 weeks. Sutures were removed at 2 weeks postoperatively and the patient was transitioned into a fracture boot at this time point. Commonly, patients will be non-weight bearing for 3 months after ORIF of a calcaneus fracture; however in this case, tricalcium phosphate cement was used to augment the posterior facet fragment fixation; therefore the patient was allowed to begin weight bearing after 6 weeks [9]. After 2 weeks in the splint, the patient was instructed to perform daily ankle range of motion exercises out of the fracture boot.

Outcome

Figure 10.3a and b demonstrates immediate postoperative radiographs. The patient has been followed in the office and his 6-month postoperative radiograph is depicted in Fig. 10.4. They demonstrate maintenance of the posterior facet reduction, fracture union, and intact implants. The patient started weight bearing as tolerated after 6 weeks of non-weight bearing and has been ambulating without pain.

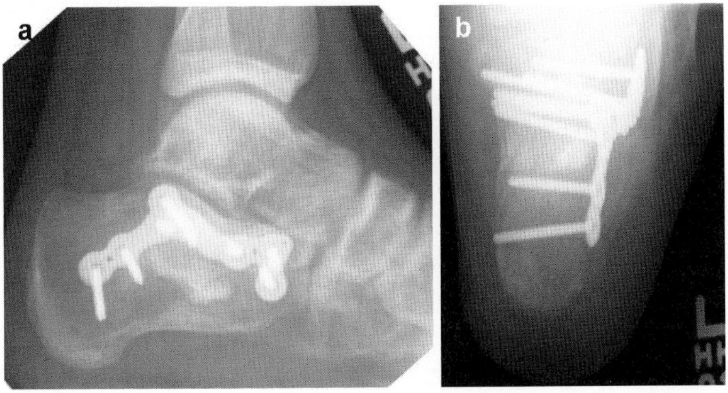

FIGURE 10.3 Immediate postoperative lateral (**a**) and Harris heel view (**b**) demonstrate anatomic heel alignment as well as restoration of the posterior articular facet and Böhler's angle

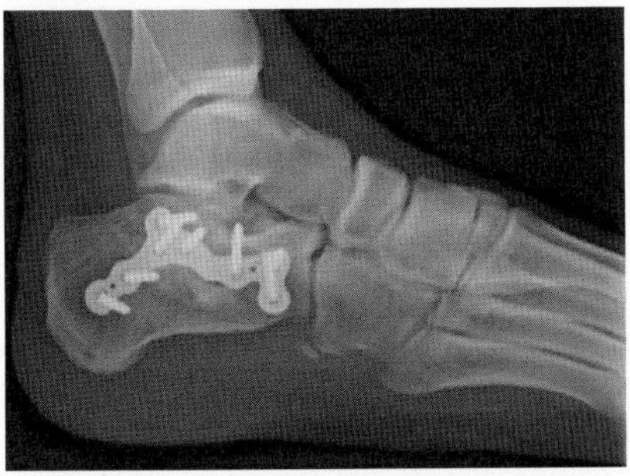

FIGURE 10.4 Six-month postoperative lateral radiograph demonstrates maintenance of the posterior facet articular reduction and fracture union

Salient Points/Pearls

- The calcaneus is the most commonly fractured tarsal bone and accounts for 1–2% of all fractures. More than 70% of all calcaneus fractures will involve the subtalar joint [10].
- Several studies have been conducted that assess both the postoperative reduction and soft tissue complications from each approach. In patients treated with the sinus tarsi approach, there is no significant difference in radiological and clinical outcomes, with a significantly decreased wound complication rate in the sinus tarsi group [2, 5, 6, 11].
- Given that the posterior tuberosity is not visualized with this approach, percutaneous reduction aids (Steinmann pins) are required to manipulate the tuberosity out of varus and to restore length [2, 6].
- Prior to plate placement one must be cognizant to clear off the lateral wall; however, care must be taken to avoid injury to the sural nerve as well as the peroneal tendons, which can be dislocated [7].
- In order to assess the posterior facet, the capsule as well as the calcaneofibular ligament must be cleared [2, 5–7].
- In highly comminuted fractures such as Sanders type IV that are not amenable to operative fixation, the limited sinus tarsi approach can be used to perform a subtalar arthrodesis [7, 12].

References

1. Benirschke SK, Kramer PA. Wound healing complications in closed and open calcaneal fractures. J Orthop Trauma. 2004;18:1–6.
2. Weber M, Lehmann O, Sagesser D, et al. Limited open reduction and internal fixation of displaced intra-articular fractures of the calcaneum. J Bone Joint Surg Br. 2008;90:1608–16.
3. Jones CP, Cohen BE. Sinus tarsi approach for calcaneal fractures. Tech Foot Ankle Surg. 2013;12:180–3.
4. Hsu AR, Anderson RB, Cohen BE. Advances in surgical management of intra-articular calcaneus fractures. JAAOS. 2015;23:399–407.

5. Kline AJ, Anderson RB, Davis WH, Jones CP, Cohen BE. Minimally invasive technique versus an extensile lateral approach for intra-articular calcaneus fractures. Foot Ankle Int. 2013;34(12):1689–94.
6. Kikuchi C, Charlton TP, Thordarson DB. Limited sinus tarsi approach for intra-articular calcaneus fractures. Foot Ankle Int. 2013;34(12):1689–94.
7. Gonzalez TA, Kwon JY. Sinus tarsi approach for calcaneus fractures. Oper Tech Orthop. 2015;23:235–41.
8. Illert T, Rammelt S, Drewes T, Grass R, Zwipp H. Stability of locking and non-locking plates in osteoporotic calcaneal fracture model. Foot Ankle Int. 2011;32(3):307–13.
9. Elsner A, Jubel A, Prokop A, Koebke J, Rehm KE, Adermahr J. Augmentation of intraarticular calcaneal fractures with injectable calcium phosphate cement: densitometry, histology, and functional outcome of 18 patients. J Foot Ankle Surg. 2005;44(5):390–5.
10. Sanders R. Displaced intra-articular fractures of the calcaneus. J Bone Joint Surg Am. 2000;82:225–50.
11. Yoe JH, Cho JH, Lee KB. Comparison of two surgical approaches for displaced intra-articular calcaneal fractures: sinus tarsi versus extensile lateral approach. BMC Musculoskelet Disord. 2015;16:63.
12. Spagnolo R, Bonalumi M, Pace F, Capitani D. Calcaneus fractures, results of the sinus tarsi approach: 4 years of experience. Eur J Orthop Surg Traumatol. 2010;20:37.

Chapter 11
Tongue-Type Calcaneus Fractures

Philip Wolinsky and Chad Beck

Case Presentation

History/Physical Exam

A healthy, active, 25-year-old male with no significant medical issues presented to our emergency department (ED) complaining of left foot pain and an inability to bear weight on the involved limb following a fall off of a second-story balcony. On physical exam he had pain to palpation over his hind foot, moderate swelling of the soft tissues over his calcaneus with significant ecchymosis, and areas of blanching skin over his posterior heel and was neurovascularly intact (Fig. 11.1). He did not have other complaints, nor any tenderness to palpation anywhere else.

P. Wolinsky, M.D. (✉)
UC Davis Medical Center, 4860 Y Street, Suite 3800,
Sacramento, CA 95817, USA
e-mail: prwolinsky@ucdavis.edu

C. Beck, M.D.
Medical College of Wisconsin, 9200 W. Wisconsin Ave,
Milwaukee, WI 53226, USA
e-mail: cjbeck@mcw.edu

N.C. Tejwani (ed.), *Fractures of the Foot and Ankle*,
DOI 10.1007/978-3-319-60456-5_11,

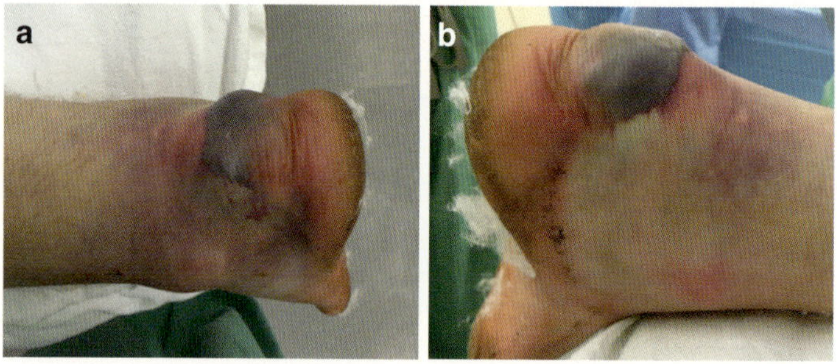

FIGURE 11.1 Soft-tissue appearance at the time of presentation to the emergency department

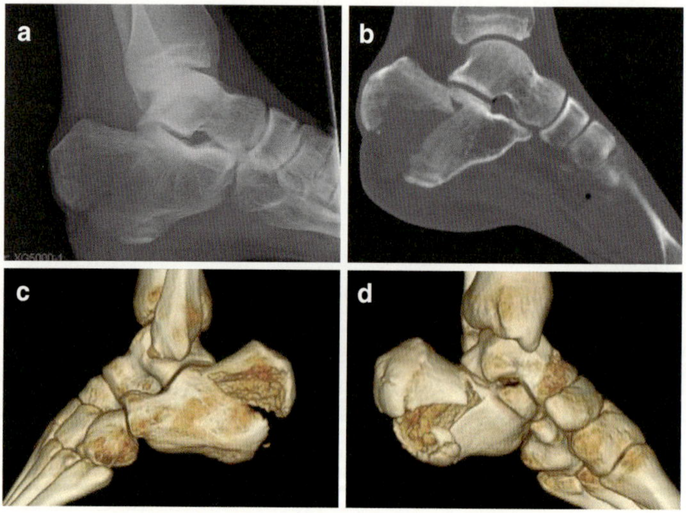

FIGURE 11.2 Plain radiographs and CT injury imaging

Radiographs

X-rays of his foot, ankle, as well as full-length tibia and fibula images (joint above and below) were obtained and showed a displaced calcaneal tuberosity tongue-type fracture. A CT scan was obtained to better delineate the injury and evaluate for any intra-articular extension into the posterior facet (Fig. 11.2).

Treatment and Timing of Surgery

This calcaneus fracture is a tongue-type injury and associated with significant soft-tissue compromise. The pressure of the displaced fragment compromising blood flow to the overlying soft tissues is reflected by the ecchymosis and skin blanching present at the time of presentation. This skin compromise requires urgent reduction and stabilization of the displaced bony fragment in the operating room to try and avoid a full-thickness soft-tissue loss. Due to this soft-tissue injury, we immediately began getting him ready to go to the operating room urgently.

In the ED, the patient was placed in a bulky Jones splint with his ankle in equinus to relax the deforming force of the Achilles tendon on the displaced fragment in the ED. This position may partly reduce the fracture and take some pressure off the soft tissues until the patient can go to the operating room. Patients with this type of fracture are typically admitted to the hospital for close monitoring of their skin envelope and brought rapidly to the operating room.

Surgical Plan

Overall Plan/Goal

Fracture reduction is the key for this case and we planned on using an escalating approach to obtain an appropriate reduction. Ideally this could be done percutaneously, but, if that were not possible we would escalate to a mini-open approach followed by a more extensile approach if needed. The key is to what is to what is necessary to take the pressure off the soft tissues while trying to protect the blood supply of the fracture fragments. In this case we were able to use small percutaneous incisions for reduction, clamp placement, and fixation.

Positioning in the Operating Room

The patient was placed in the prone position on a radiolucent foot extension so C-arm imaging cold be used intraoperatively, and both sides of the calcaneus are accessible.

The patient's foot was positioned at the end of the table to help facilitate access to the foot and for proper imaging. Either blankets or "bone foam" can be used to elevate the injured extremity above the other to facilitate obtaining a lateral image. This setup facilitates access to the posterior aspect of the patient's foot for reduction and fixation of the fracture. Alternatively, the lateral position could be used, but makes access to the medial side of the foot difficult if needed during the procedure.

Fracture Reduction

We began by unroofing and debriding the skin blisters. Fluoroscopy was then used to help plan our incisions by localizing and marking the positions of the fracture line and both fragments. The foot plantar-flexed to see how much that maneuver reduced the displaced tuberosity fragment. Once the fragments were closer together we used a combination of palpation and fluoroscopy to determine the positions of the superior and inferior aspects of the calcaneal tuberosity. The tines of a large Weber clamp were placed where we thought they would clamp the fragments together and their positions checked using a lateral fluoroscopic image prior to making stab incisions. Four 1-cm stab incisions were then made so we could place the tines of two large Weber clamps on the medial and lateral sides of the calcaneus to reduce and compress the fracture fragments. The clamps were positioned so they did not place any pressure on the already compromised soft tissues. The first time we clamped the fracture together we caused skin puckering on the medial side where soft tissue was trapped within the fracture site. After unclamping we made a small incision over this area and used an elevator to sweep the soft tissues out the fracture site. We were then able to re-clamp the fracture site without any soft tissues being trapped within the fracture site. We then obtained lateral and Harris heel views to check our reduction. 1.6 mm K-wires were then placed to help hold the reduction.

Fracture Fixation

Once we were satisfied with our reduction we placed three 3.2 mm guide wires for 6.5 mm cannulated screws from superior to inferior and perpendicular to the fracture line. We prefer to use larger fixation for fixation of the calcaneal tuberosity fixation if the size of the fragments allows this to counteract the strong pull of the Achilles tendon; however, successful treatment using screws as small as 2.7 mm has been described. Once we verified that the guide wires were in the proper positions on lateral and Harris axial heel views, we placed the appropriate length 6.5 mm cannulated screws through stab wounds (Fig. 11.3). We used a washer on one screw to aid in fixation and prevent intrusion of the screw into the tuberosity. Screw "traffic" prevented the use of a washer on all three screws. The stab incisions were closed with nylon sutures, Silvadene and Xeroform were placed over the unroofed blisters, and the patient was splinted in plantar flexion to protect the fixation/reduction.

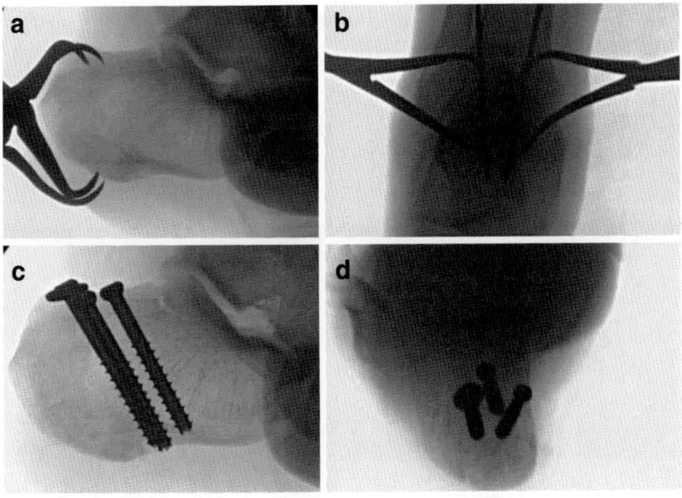

Figure 11.3 Intraoperative imaging

Postoperative Plan

A short leg posterior splint with a stirrup was placed in the operating room with the patient in their "resting" equinus position. Post-discharge follow-up timing is dependent on the condition of the skin at the time of discharge. At a minimum the patient is seen within 2 weeks for a skin check and suture removal. If the skin is questionable the patient will return sooner. If the fixation was felt to be "good" at the time of surgery (good bone and good "bite") and the soft tissues are well healed at 2-week postoperative check, we start the patient on gentle ankle range of motion at that time. If the fixation was less than optimal or the soft tissues need more "rest" we will slowly correct the equinus over the first 8 weeks postoperatively with either serial casting (never if the skin is compromised and/or requires wound care) or a CAM boot with decreasing heel lifts. The patient is kept toe touch weight bearing for the first 8 weeks.

At 8 weeks a radiograph is obtained (Fig. 11.4) and weight bearing is progressed over the next 4 weeks from toe touch to weight bearing as tolerated with pain being the limiting factor. At 3 months postoperative if the patients have been able to progress to full weight bearing and are comfortable, and X-rays show appropriate healing, we will allow the patient to begin strengthening exercises.

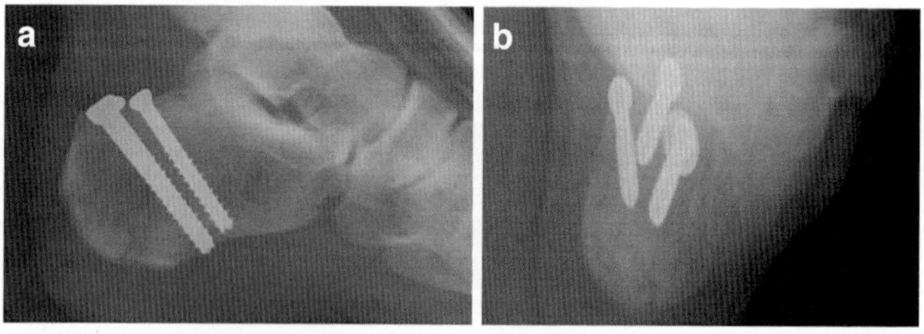

FIGURE 11.4 Postoperative plain radiographs

Salient Points/Pearls

- This fracture is one of the few remaining true orthopedic emergencies. The condition of the soft-tissue envelope is the key factor that dictates the urgency of treatment. Soft-tissues necrosis can quickly develop due to the blood supply compromise caused by direct pressure of the displaced fragment. Interposed soft tissues may block any provisional reduction that can be obtained with plantarflexion. Soft-tissue compromise has been seen in up to 21% of patients with tongue-type injuries [1, 2].
- Surgical approaches that have been used to address this fracture pattern include posteromedial, posterolateral, extensile lateral, sinus tarsi, direct posterior, and percutaneous approaches. Authors recommend allowing the soft-tissue envelope and the comfort of the surgeon to dictate which technique(s) is needed to obtain fracture reduction and fixation. Surgery is typically performed using either the prone or the lateral position. Fixation options include percutaneous screw placement to plate fixation with more open approaches [1–4].
- The most described reduction maneuver for tongue-type fractures is the Essex-Lopresti maneuver. This involves percutaneously placing K-wires/Steinmann pins into the proximally displaced fragment parallel to the fracture line. The mid foot is the held in one hand and plantarflexed. Simultaneously a proximal to distal force is placed through the wires close down the fracture site. This is held is this position until provisional fixation can be achieved. This method was seen to give an accurate reduction in up to 88% of the cases [2, 3].
- The primary deforming force on the calcaneal tuberosity is the insertion of the Achilles tendon. This needs to be considered for any possible preexisting contractures. Some authors have advocated gastrocnemius recession or tendo-achilles lengthening to help reduce the deforming force on fracture fixation [4].

References

1. Gardner MJ, Nork SE, Barei DP, Kramer PA, Sangeorzan BJ, Benirschke SK. Secondary soft tissue compromise in tongue-type calcaneus fractures. J Orthop Trauma. 2008;22(7):439–45. doi:10.1097/BOT.0b013e31817ace7e.
2. Letournel E. Open treatment of acute calcaneal fractures. Clin Orthop Relat Res. 1993;290:60–7.
3. Tornetta P. The Essex-Lopresti reduction for calcaneal fractures revisited. J Orthop Trauma. 1998;12(7):469–73.
4. Banerjee R, Chao JC, Taylor R, Siddiqui A. Management of calcaneal tuberosity fractures. J Am Acad Orthop Surg. 2012;20(4):253–8. doi:10.5435/JAAOS-20-04-253.

Chapter 12
Cuboid and Nutcracker Fractures

Daniel Segina and Ryan Wilson

Case Presentation

The case presentation is a 21-year-old male involved in a motor vehicle collision as a restrained driver. He reported no loss of consciousness and arrived via helicopter in full backboard and cervical spine immobilization. ATLS protocol was initiated and the patient was noted to be hemodynamically stable. The patient was awake, alert, and oriented. He complained of right foot and right lower leg pain. There was an obvious deformity to his right lower extremity with exposed bone. Pulses were present via Doppler examination with gross sensation intact to light touch. The open wound over his mid-tibia was dressed with a saline-soaked sterile gauze bandage, and well-padded short leg splint was applied.

D. Segina, M.D. (✉)
Department of Orthopaedic Surgery,
Holmes Regional Medical Center, Melbourne, FL 32901, USA
e-mail: dsegina@cfl.rr.com

R. Wilson, P.A.-C., M.P.A.S.
Department of Orthopaedics, Holmes Regional Medical Center,
Melbourne, FL 32901, USA

N.C. Tejwani (ed.), *Fractures of the Foot and Ankle*,
DOI 10.1007/978-3-319-60456-5_12,

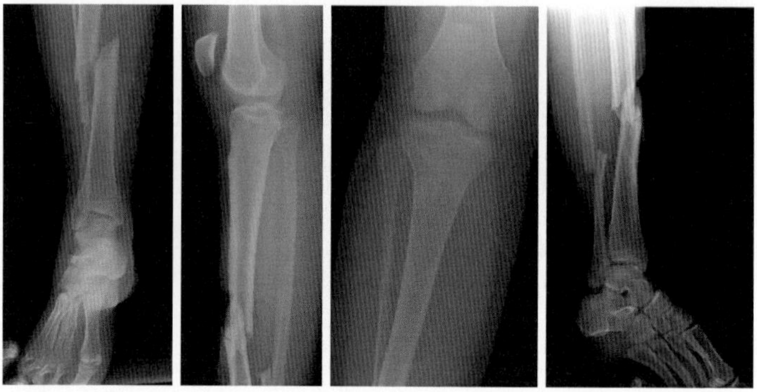

FIGURE 12.1 AP and lateral injury radiographs of the right tibia and right foot

Injury Films

AP and lateral plain film radiographs of the right lower extremity, foot, and ankle demonstrated fractures of the tibia and fibula, first through third metatarsals, and navicular (Fig. 12.1). A CT scan with two-dimensional and three-dimensional reformats was performed which confirmed fractures observed on plain film, in addition to fractures of the cuboid and first metatarsal base (Figs. 12.2 and 12.3).

Treatment and Timing of Surgery

After administration of appropriate prophylactic antibiotics, the patient was taken to the operating room for emergent treatment of his open tibia and fibula fractures. After tibial stabilization, stress radiographs were obtained to further assess the foot injury. First tarsal-metatarsal joint instability was noted along with an avulsion fracture of the base of the second metatarsal (Fig. 12.4). Excessive swelling of the foot

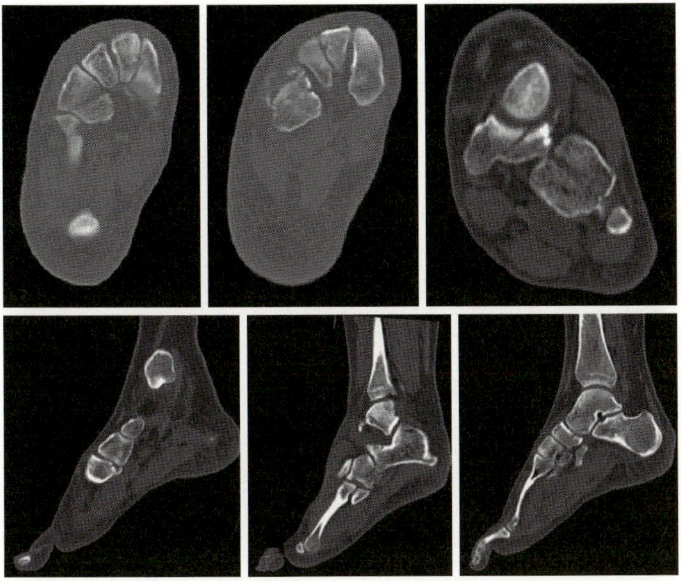

FIGURE 12.2 Axial, coronal, and sagittal reformats of the right foot

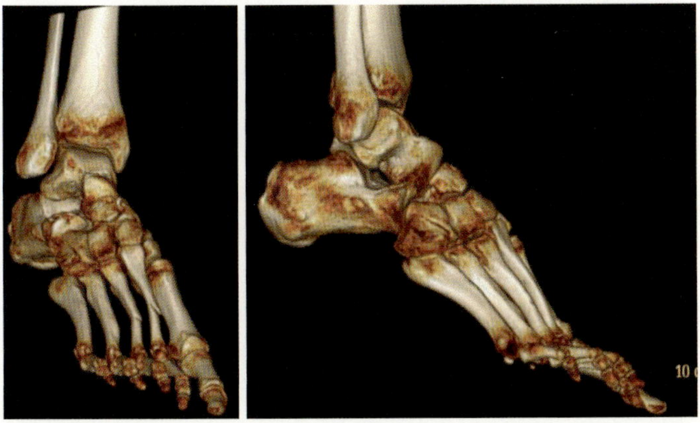

FIGURE 12.3 Three-dimensional reformats of the right foot

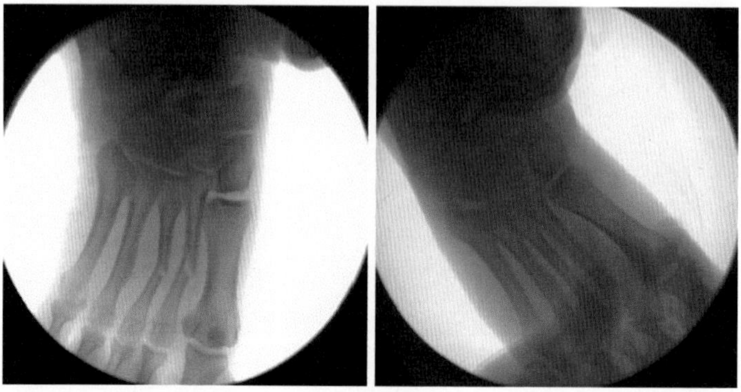

FIGURE 12.4 Intraoperative stress radiographs

was present and therefore it was planned to perform delayed reconstruction of the foot injuries. Postoperatively, the patient was placed into a well-padded posterior splint for soft-tissue immobilization. The patient had significant foot and ankle edema, which precluded surgical intervention at the primary hospital admission. He was discharged to home and then seen in the outpatient office 7 days later to assess edema. Once his edema had resolved and the soft tissues were amenable to surgical dissection, he was electively scheduled for repair of his right-foot injury.

Surgical Tact

Position

Supine on a radiolucent operating table with a rolled sheet bump under the ipsilateral hip and fluoroscopy from the contralateral side of the table. The operative leg had an unsterile tourniquet placed prior to draping and a sterile radiolucent padded triangle was placed behind the knee for optimal positioning of the foot and relaxation of the gastrocnemius soleus (Fig. 12.5). Appropriate antibiotic prophylaxis was delivered within 60 mins of incision and a surgical time-out was performed.

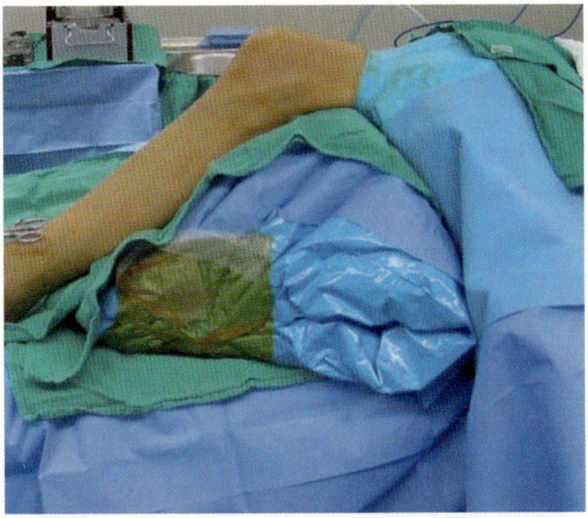

FIGURE 12.5 Limb position with padded triangular wedge

Approach

Due to combined medial and lateral columnar injuries, a dual-incision approach was utilized. This encompassed a dorsal medial utility incision as well as a lateral incision allowing for surgical visualization of the first and second tarsometatarsal junction, navicular injury, as well as lateral column/cuboid injury.

Fracture Reduction and Fixation (Medial Column)

Reconstruction began with medial column restoration. Direct exposure of the entire medial column provided for anatomical reduction and safe hardware placement. Reconstruction began by addressing the first metatarsal injury. Direct visualization of the joint is mandatory to avoid medial columnar mal-reduction. Retrograde screw fixation from the base of the first metatarsal into the medial cuneiform was utilized and provided for adequate stabilization.

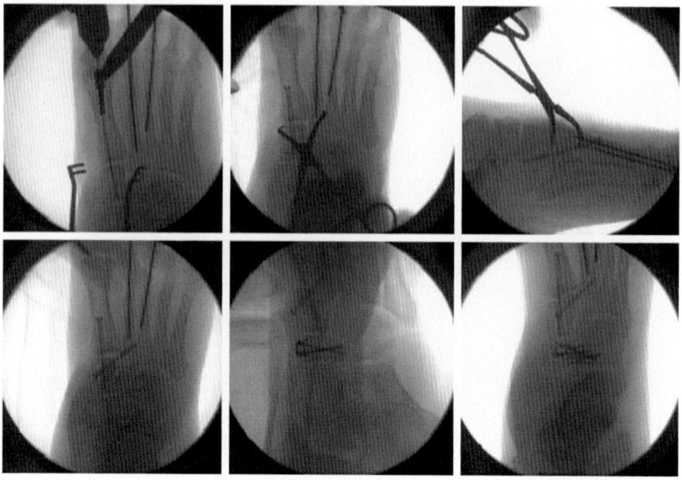

FIGURE 12.6 Intraoperative views of the medial column reconstruction

Adequacy of the reduction was assessed with both direct visualization and adjuvant fluoroscopy. After fixation of the first tarsometatarsal injury, the second metatarsal base/Lisfranc joint complex was evaluated to assess anatomical alignment. Finally, reconstruction of the medial column addressed the navicular injury. Direct exposure of the navicular provided for anatomical reduction and safe hardware placement (Fig. 12.6).

Fracture Reduction and Fixation (Lateral Column)

Attention was then focused on the lateral column injury focusing on the cuboid. A linear incision was made in line with the fourth metatarsal and extended proximally to ensure adequate visualization of the cuboid (Fig. 12.7). Subcutaneous branches of the superficial peroneal nerve are commonly seen after skin incision and should be gently dissected

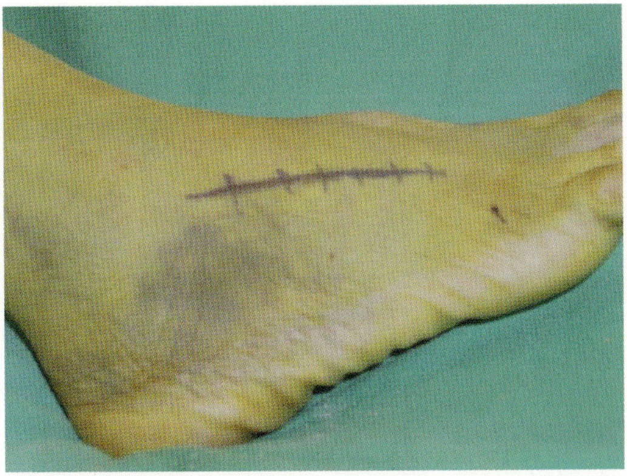

FIGURE 12.7 Surgical approach

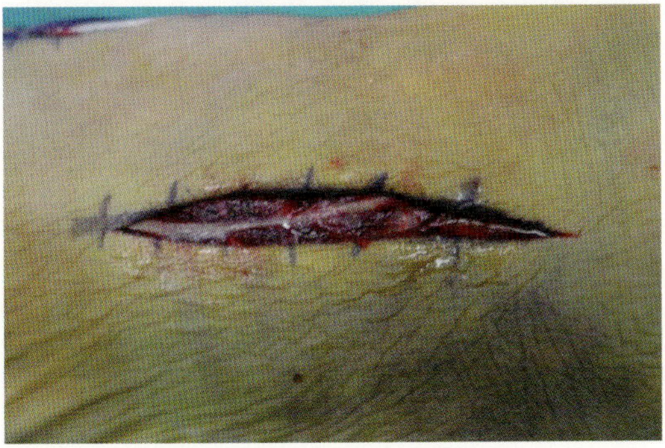

FIGURE 12.8 Superficial peroneal nerve branch

(Fig. 12.8). The interval between the peroneus tertius and peroneus brevis is exploited to reveal the underlying lateral wall of the cuboid. Further dissection proximally reveals the inferior aspect of the extensor digitorum brevis muscle belly. This was elevated as a full-thickness flap from the lateral cuboid (Fig. 12.9). Next, the articulations at the calcaneal cuboid and cuboid metatarsal joints were directly visualized (Fig. 12.10). Articular impaction was addressed with

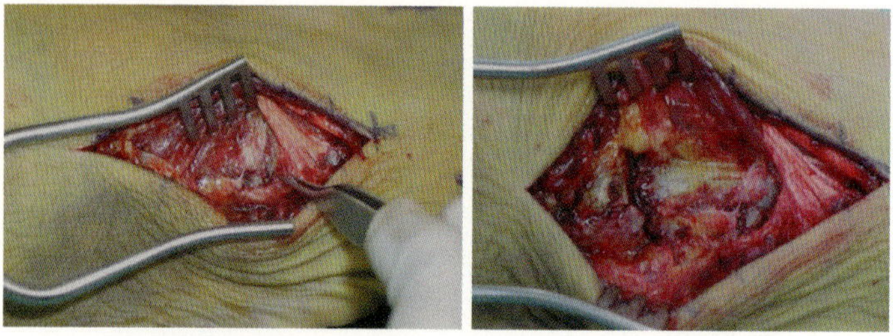

FIGURE 12.9 Deep dissection with cuboid exposure

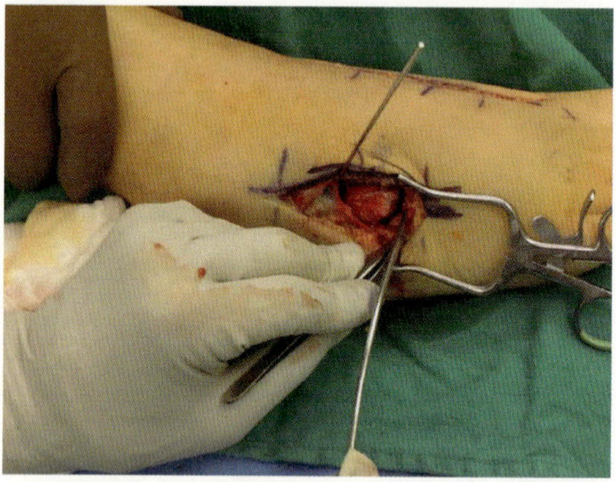

FIGURE 12.10 Deep exposure with visualization of the cuboid metatarsal articulation

mobilization of the lateral cuboid cortical surface and elevation of the depressed articular segments to produce a congruent articular surface (Fig. 12.11). Any bone void should be addressed with supplemental graft material (i.e., allograft bone graft) and temporary K-wire fixation is placed to maintain the reduction. Definitive stabilization was accomplished with small fragment plate fixation. Contouring is usually necessary to ensure appropriate screw placement/trajectory and minimize hardware prominence. Newer anatomically

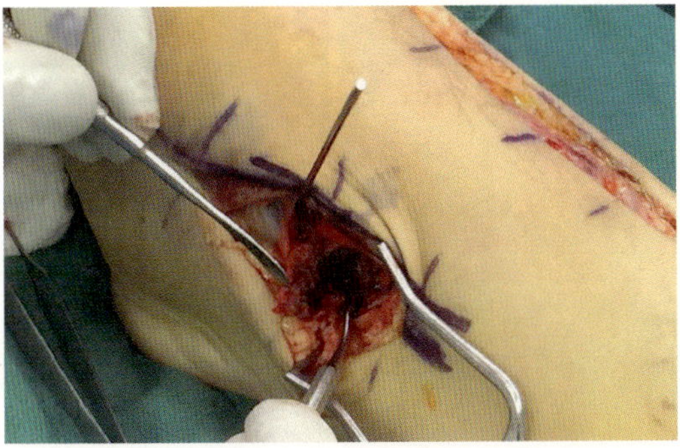

FIGURE 12.11 Exposure of cuboid articular impaction

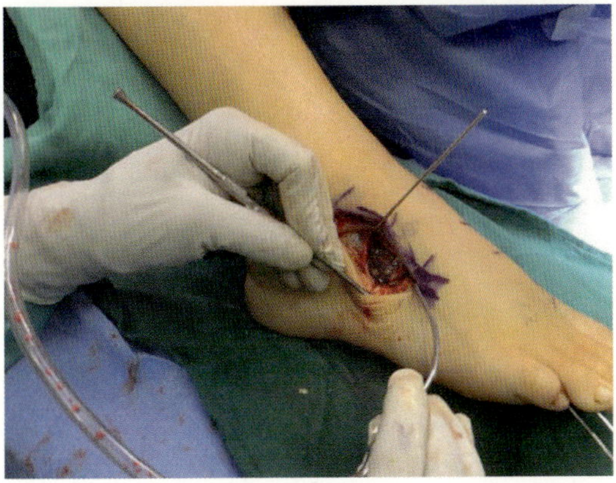

FIGURE 12.12 Placement of anatomically contoured cuboid plate

contoured plates may be beneficial for certain fracture patterns. Additionally, angular stable screw fixation may be warranted for patients with severe comminution or osteoporotic bone (Fig. 12.12).

After definitive fixation, articular surfaces were inspected for congruency and stability. Position of the hardware was assessed with the use of intraoperative fluoroscopic imaging (Fig. 12.13).

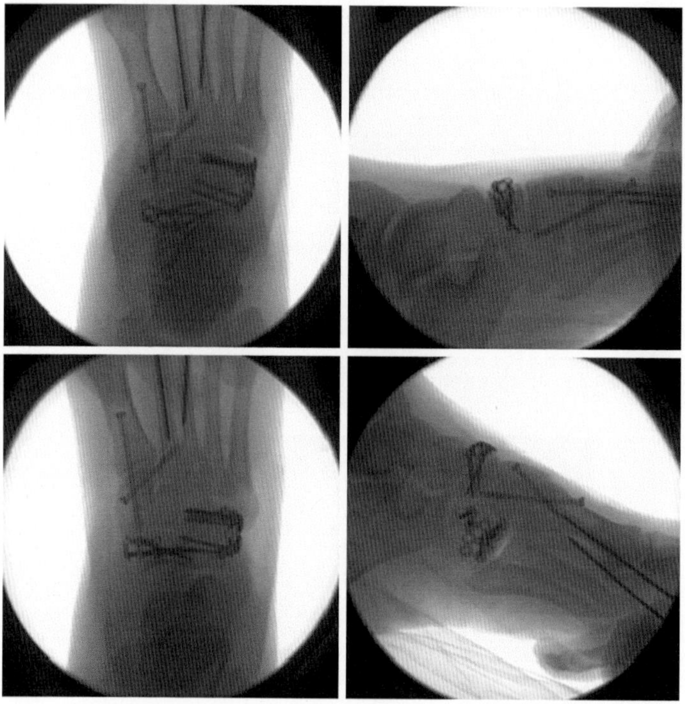

FIGURE 12.13 Final intraoperative images

Postoperative Plan

After the surgical incisions were dressed sterile, a well-padded short-leg posterior splint was applied for positional comfort and soft-tissue immobilization. Toes were left exposed to allow for adequate postoperative neurocirculatory evaluations. The patient was given appropriate prophylactic antibiotics for 24 h postoperatively. Deep venous thromboembolism prophylaxis is ideally based upon risk assessment, but at a minimum, should include mechanical compression to the contralateral limb.

Outcome

The patient was seen in follow-up in the outpatient office for suture removal 10 days post-definitive repair and physical therapy without weight bearing was initiated. The therapy protocol focused on edema control and range-of-motion exercises to prevent equinus contracture. Serial radiographs were obtained at 6-week intervals for 3 months. Temporary K-wire fixation was discontinued at 6 weeks postoperatively.

Aquatic therapy was initiated at 6 weeks with full weight bearing allowed to begin at 10 weeks. Aggressive formal and self-directed physical therapy continued until 8 months post-injury. At that time, radiographs revealed healed fractures of the tibia, fibula, midfoot, and forefoot.

Following a routine protocol, screw removal was performed 9 months post-injury (Fig. 12.14). Final functional outcome included minimal pain, full return to work as a construction worker, and normal gait.

Salient Points/Pearls

- Fractures of the cuboid present a diagnostic dilemma due to vague clinical symptoms and complex osteology. Clinical suspicion should always be present with a combination of midfoot swelling, ecchymosis, and pain.
- Cuboid fractures rarely occur in isolation; therefore the concern always exists for associated injuries [1–4]. Plain-film oblique radiographs help with the initial assessment of a potential injury. CT evaluation with 2D and 3D reformats is mandatory to accurately assess the overall cuboid architecture as well as determine frequently associated additional injuries [1].
- Stress radiographs can help determine subtle instabilities and are recommended if the clinical opportunities arise (Fig. 12.4).

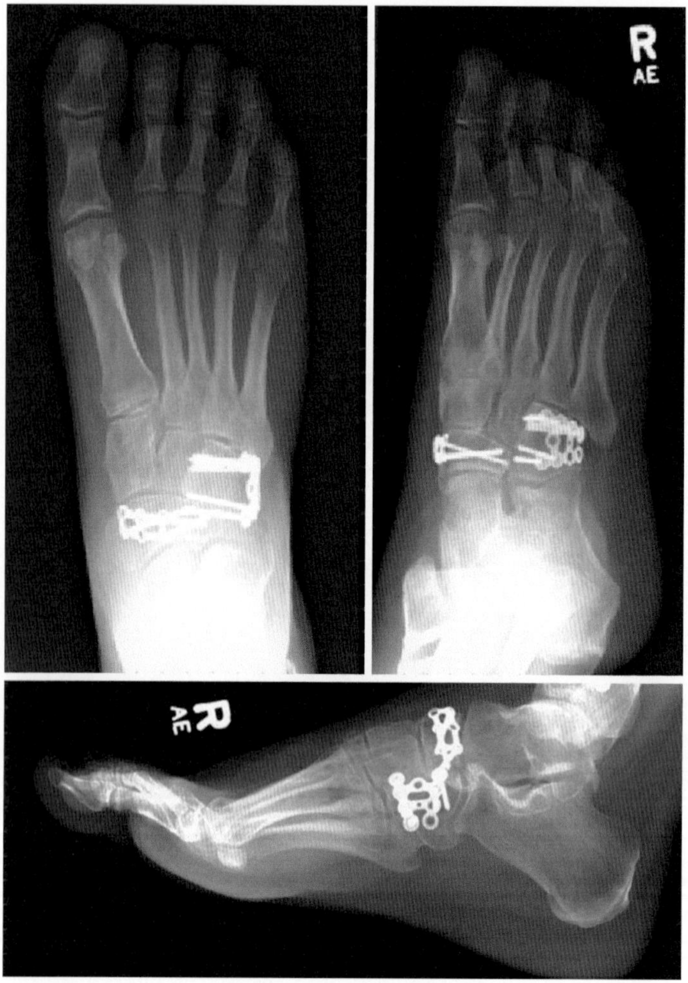

FIGURE 12.14 Final plain films 9 months post-op

- The timing of fixation is dependent upon soft-tissue swelling resolution. Columnar external fixation or medullary K-wires can provide temporary stabilization while maintaining length and assisting in soft-tissue swelling resolution (Fig. 12.15).

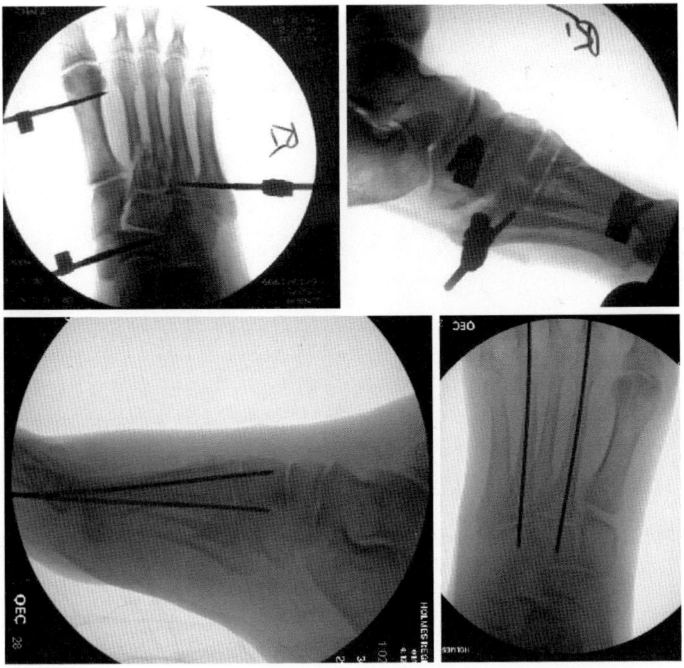

FIGURE 12.15 Temporary fixation with either external fixation or temporary K-wires

- Pending compartment syndrome is always a concern. Mechanism of injury combined with physical examination and compartment pressure measurements all contribute to the diagnosis. Timely temporizing stabilization, combined with fascial release, is the usual treatment. Fascial release can be achieved through larger medial and lateral incisions or multiple small (pie crust) incisions (Fig. 12.16). Either method needs to take into account future surgical approaches to help avoid skin compromise.
- Frequently, multiple incisions/approaches are needed to address the full constellation of injuries. Careful planning is used to maximize injury visualization and preserve skin bridges to avoid postoperative wound issues.

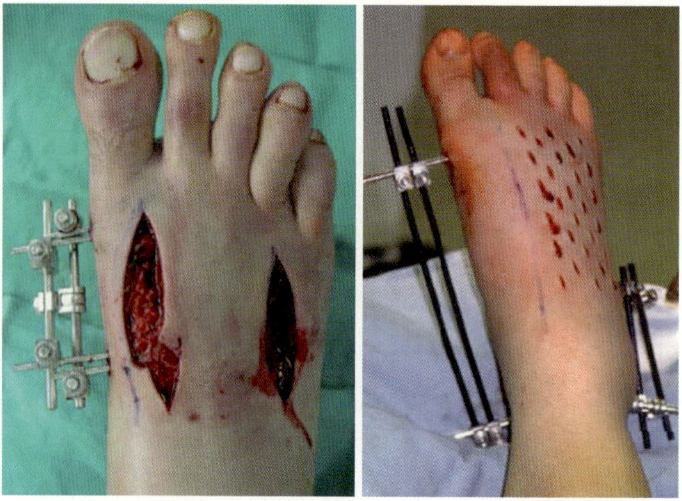

FIGURE 12.16 Fasciotomy incisions

- If associated injuries are present, surgical reconstruction usually begins medially, with restoration of the medial column and/or first–third tarsal-metatarsal joints. Screw fixation remains the preferred stabilization technique with plate fixation occasionally utilized for significant comminution or column substitution. Retrograde medullary K-wire stabilization can be useful for stabilization while helping to avoid soft-tissue disruption (Fig. 12.17).
- Definitive stabilization of the cuboid injury mandates direct visualization via an open exposure. A generous incision is made in line with the fourth metatarsal, allowing for calcaneal cuboid and cuboid metatarsal articular assessment. Sural and superficial peroneal nerve branches are carefully mobilized away from the operative approach. The interval between the peroneus tertius and peroneus brevis is utilized along with full-thickness elevation of the extensor digitorum brevis muscle belly [1–3].
- A bone void filler should be readily available to support corrected articular impaction.

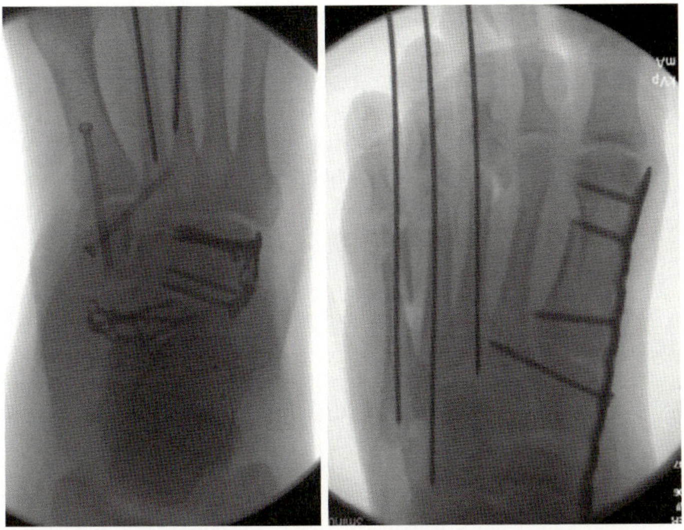

FIGURE 12.17 Temporary K-wire stabilization

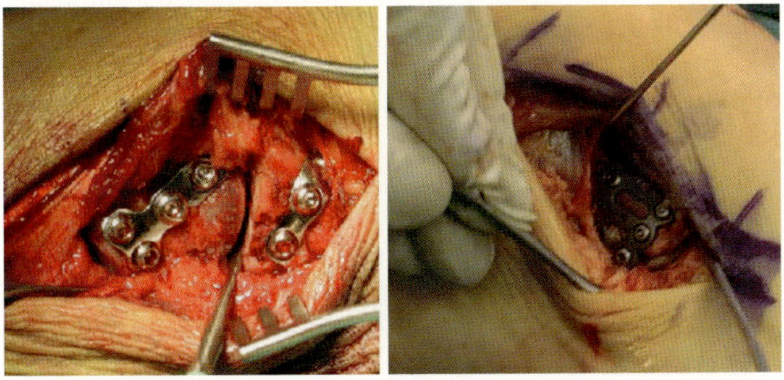

FIGURE 12.18 Plate fixation options

- Plate fixation is frequently chosen to support the restored cuboid anatomy and maintain graft containment. Newer, anatomically contoured small fragment plates with locking screw options may enhance surgical repair. However, the potential clinical benefit should be weighed against the added cost (Fig. 12.18).

- Postoperative protocol needs to take into account the frequently encountered constellation of injuries. Six to eight weeks of strict non-weight bearing followed by 4–6 weeks of protected weight bearing allows adequate healing time for both the osseous and ligamentous injuries (author's preferred method). The inclusion of aquatic exercises may allow for earlier weight bearing and enhance the recovery process.

References

1. Borelli J, De S, VanPelt M. Fractures of the cuboid. JAAOS. 2012;20(7):472–7.
2. Sangeorzan BJ, Swiontkowski MF. Displaced fractures of the cuboid. J Bone Joint Surg Br. 1990;72(3):376–8.
3. Weber M, Locher S. Reconstruction of the cuboid in compression fractures: short to midterm results in 12 patients. Foot Ankle Int. 2002;23(11):1008–13.
4. Hermel MB, Gershon-Cohen J. The nutcracker fracture of the cuboid by indirect violence. Radiology. 1953;60(6):850–4.

Chapter 13
Navicular Fractures

Mark Ayoub and David Polonet

Case Presentation #1

A 45-year-old male unrestrained driver in a motor vehicle collision sustained a closed fracture-dislocation of the right navicular. Associated injuries included a posterior ipsilateral hip dislocation. His medical history included prior knee surgery and chronic back pain and anxiety. He was using Klonopin and oxycodone prior to this injury.

Injury Films

AP, lateral, and oblique radiographs of the foot and a CT scan were obtained (Figs. 13.1 and 13.2).

M. Ayoub, M.D.
Department of Orthopaedic Surgery, Rutgers-Robert Wood Johnson University Hospital, New Brunswick, NJ 08903-0019, USA

D. Polonet, M.D. (✉)
Department of Orthopaedic Surgery, Jersey Shore University Medical Center, Wall, NJ 07753, USA
e-mail: dpolonet@yahoo.com

N.C. Tejwani (ed.), *Fractures of the Foot and Ankle*,
DOI 10.1007/978-3-319-60456-5_13,

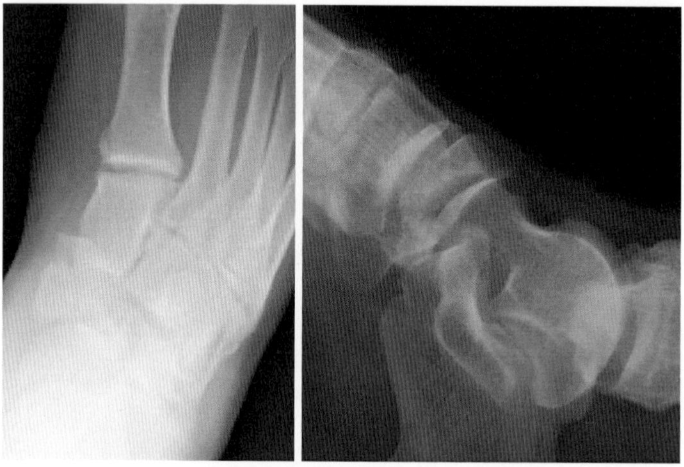

FIGURE 13.1 AP and lateral radiographs showing a fracture-dislocation of the right navicular

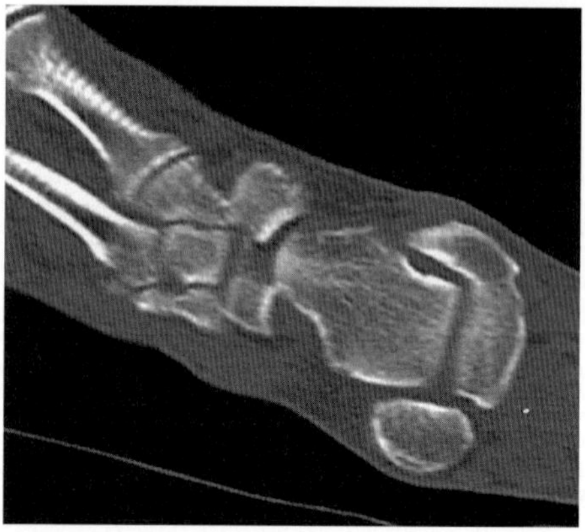

FIGURE 13.2 Axial CT cut illustrating large displaced dorsomedial fragment of the navicular

Treatment and Timing of Surgery

Following examination and radiographic analysis of the injury, the hip dislocation was reduced. It was noted that the navicular dislocation was unable to be maintained in a reduced position. The patient was taken urgently to the operating room for open reduction internal fixation due to tenting of the skin and concern for skin necrosis.

Surgical Tact

Position

The patient was placed on the operating table in the supine position, with a thigh tourniquet. Once draped to the level of the tourniquet, the knee was flexed over a radiolucent triangle and the foot slightly elevated with respect to the opposite lower extremity, allowing for unimpeded lateral fluoroscopic views.

Approach

The tourniquet was not inflated. A dorsomedial incision was made extending from the distal talus to the distal medial cuneiform. Deep exposure involved retraction of the dorsalis pedis artery and deep peroneal nerve.

Fracture Reduction and Fixation

Bone fragments were identified, cleaned, and reduced using plantar pressure and manual distraction. Two main fragments across the central aspect of the navicular were held using a bone reduction forceps. This was then secured using a smooth Kirschner wire and two partially threaded cannulated 4.0-mm cancellous screws were placed from medial to lateral, one dorsal and the other plantar. These navicular screws were placed through two small medial stab incisions. The navicular was then pinned from the medial and intermediate cuneiform, through the navicular, into the talus with two smooth 2.0-mm Kirschner wires to provide additional stability to the medial column (Fig. 13.3). The wound was closed, after tourniquet release and saline irrigation, in layers with 2-0 Vicryl and 3-0 nylon sutures.

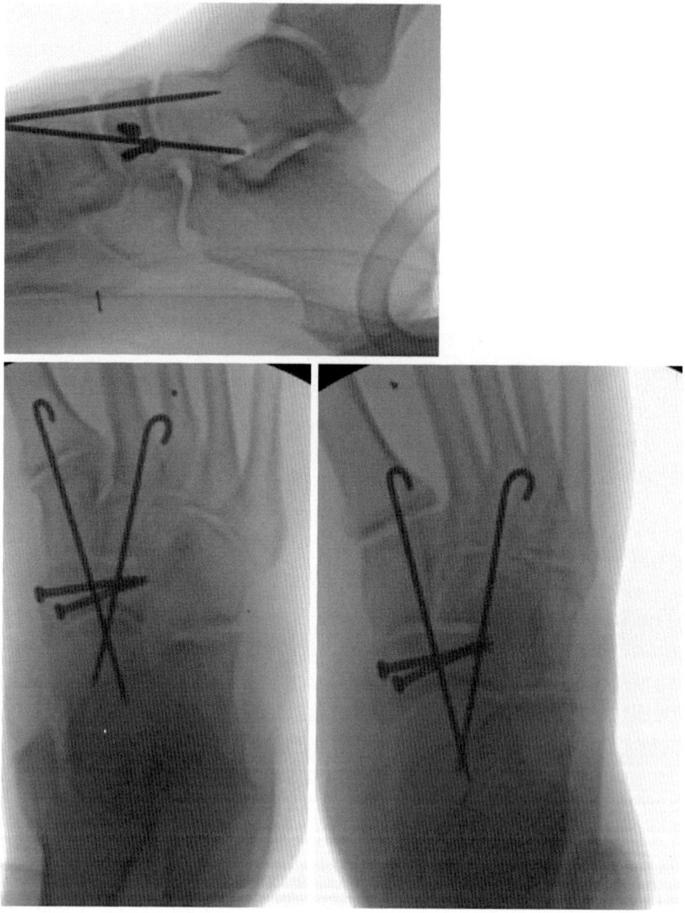

FIGURE 13.3 Postoperative radiographs showing fixation of the navicular and medial column

Postoperative Plan

An AO splint was applied. Antibiotics were maintained for 24 h perioperatively. The patient was instructed to maintain foot-flat touchdown weight bearing for 10 weeks. Elevation to heart level was instructed. The sutures were removed at 2 weeks, and the patient was placed into a removable cam-walker boot. Ankle and toe range-of-motion exercises

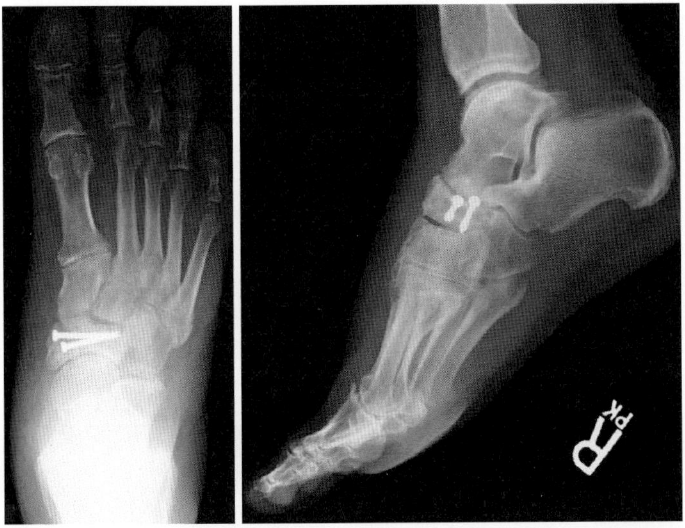

FIGURE 13.4 Final X-rays, 1 year post-injury

were initiated. Pins were removed at 4 weeks without re-subluxation.

Outcome

The patient had multifocal post-injury pain, although his midfoot pain was mild. His primary complaint regarding his foot was swelling. He had diminished sensation in his saphenous nerve distribution that slowly improved. He returned to work 6 months post-injury. He was discharged from care 1 year post-injury. Final X-rays are shown (Fig. 13.4).

Case Presentation #2

A 34-year-old male involved in a motorcycle collision presented complaining of right-foot pain. No other complaints were noted. He was stable hemodynamically, and ATLS-based assessment revealed no other sites of injury. Skin was intact, with mild swelling over the midfoot. No neurovascular compromise was seen.

Injury Films

Radiographs and a CT were obtained (Figs. 13.5 and 13.6). 3D reconstruction images were created from CT data showing a comminuted navicular (Fig. 13.7).

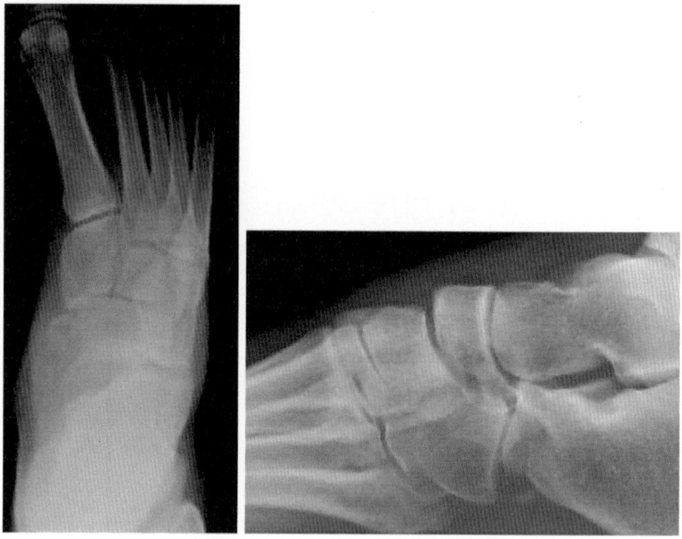

FIGURE 13.5 AP, oblique, and lateral radiographs showing a comminuted navicular fracture

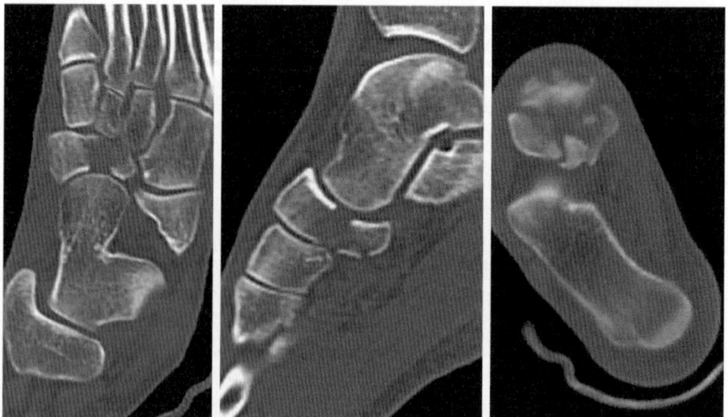

FIGURE 13.6 Axial, sagittal, and coronal CT cuts

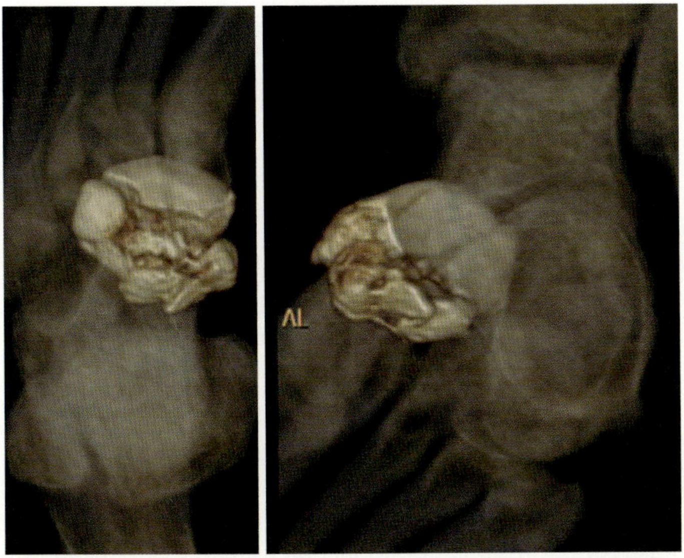

FIGURE 13.7 3D reconstruction of the navicular illustrating extensive plantar comminution

Treatment and Timing of Surgery

The patient was indicated for surgery and consent obtained. While surgery was not deemed urgent or emergent, the foot was suitable for surgery the same day and swelling was mild. The dedicated orthopedic trauma operating room schedule allowed for his surgical care to be completed that day. He was brought to the operating room within 4 h of presentation.

Surgical Tact

Position and Approach

Position was supine with the radiolucent triangle. Tourniquet was loosely applied but not inflated. Dual incisions, dorsal and medial, were used to approach the fracture. The dorsal incision was in line with the third ray, centered over the navicular. Exposure required mobilization of a superficial peroneal nerve branch. Two main fragments, one large dorsal medial fragment and a lateral fragment, were identified after tendons were retracted medially and the retinaculum and capsule incised. The second (medial) incision extended from the talonavicular joint to the medial cuneiform. The tibialis anterior tendon was identified and retracted anteriorly. A small distractor was placed on the medial side of the foot to assist with exposure. This was done by placing a 3-mm Schanz pin into the first metatarsal base and a second pin into the talar neck. The navicular was secondarily distracted using a lamina spreader to allow fragment mobilization and visualization of the plantar surface of the navicular.

Fracture Reduction and Fixation

Both windows were exploited simultaneously. The fracture was reduced from lateral to medial using the talar head as a template to reduce the articular surface. Temporary Kirschner wires were replaced with fragment-specific 2.4-mm plates and screws. Adjacent joint instability was addressed with trans-articular screws and spanning plates (Fig. 13.8).

Postoperative Plan

An AO splint was applied. Antibiotics were maintained for 24 h perioperatively. The patient was instructed to maintain foot-flat touchdown weight bearing for 10 weeks. Elevation to heart level was instructed. The sutures were removed at 2 weeks, and the patient was placed into a removable cam-walker boot. Ankle and toe range-of-motion exercises were initiated.

Outcome

While there was minimal complaint of pain, stiffness and swelling were reported. It was recommended that trans-articular plates be electively removed 6 months postoperatively; however, the patient declined any further surgery. Final X-rays are shown at 6 months (Fig. 13.9).

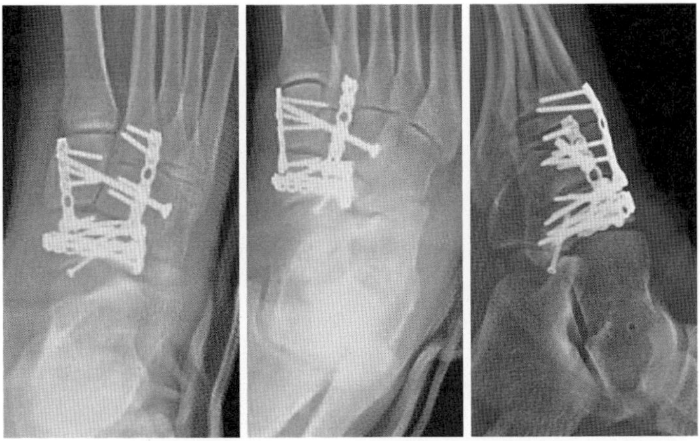

FIGURE 13.8 Postoperative radiographs. Fixation of the navicular is achieved using a 2.4-mm cannulated screw and a 2.4-mm T-plate. Another 2.4-mm T-plate spans the naviculocuneiform joint to provide additional stability to the medial column, and a 3.5-mm screw is used to fixate the medial, middle, and lateral cuneiforms. Lastly, an additional 2.4-mm T-plate spans the naviculocuneiform-second metatarsal joints

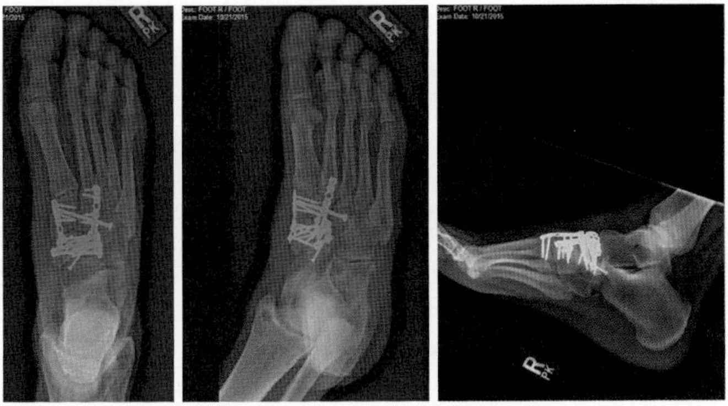

FIGURE 13.9 X-rays at 6 months postoperatively

Salient Points/Pearls

- A high index of suspicion for concomitant injury to the ipsilateral midfoot and hindfoot must be maintained. Associated injury to the cuboid or intercuneiform ligaments must be ruled out.
- The talar articular surface of the navicular has a concave shape. Screws at this location must be angled distally into the navicular to avoid joint penetration [1].
- The talonavicular joint is the most mobile midfoot joint and fusion results in degeneration of the subtalar and calcaneocuboid joints [1–4].
- The central area of the navicular is a watershed area that makes it more susceptible to avascular necrosis, nonunion, and stress fractures [5, 6].
- A 2-incision approach, utilizing both dorsal and medial intervals, can be used in more complex fracture patterns with comminution. Caution should be taken to protect the superficial peroneal nerve as well as the deep peroneal nerve with the more lateral window.
- Use of medially applied external fixator to the first metatarsal and medial talar neck can assist with exposure of the navicular as well as in restoring the length of the medial column [2].
- In fractures with comminution, strong consideration should be given to plate and screw constructs [1, 7, 8].
- Alternative or supplemental treatment options such as primary arthrodesis of the naviculocuneiform joints, primary talonavicular/medial column arthrodesis, application of a spanning external fixator, delayed reconstruction, and temporary medial column bridge plating should be considered in cases with severe comminution not amenable to open reduction internal fixation [2, 4, 9].

References

1. Cronier P, Frin JM, Steiger V, Bigorre N, Talha A. Internal fixation of complex fractures of the tarsal navicular with locking plates. A report of 10 cases. Orthop Traumatol Surg Res. 2013;99 (4 Suppl):S241–9.
2. Ramadorai MU, Beuchel MW, Sangeorzan BJ. Fractures and dislocations of the tarsal navicular. J Am Acad Orthop Surg. 2016;24(6):379–89.
3. Sanders R, Fortin P, DiPasquale T, et al. Operative treatment in 120 displaced intraarticular calcaneal fractures. Results using a prognostic computed tomography scan classification. Clin Orthop. 1993;290:87–95.
4. Astion DJ, Deland JT, Otis JC, Kenneally S. Motion of the hindfoot after simulated arthrodesis. J Bone Joint Surg Am. 1997;79(2):241–6.
5. Rosenbaum AJ, Uhl RL, DiPreta JA. Acute fractures of the tarsal navicular. Orthopedics. 2014;37(8):541–6.
6. Golano P, Farinas O, Saenz I. The anatomy of the navicular and periarticular structures. Foot Ankle Clin. 2004;9:1–23.
7. Richter M, Wippermann B, Krettek C, Schratt HE, Hufner T, Thermann H. Fractures and fracture dislocations of the midfoot: occurrence, causes and long-term results. Foot Ankle Int. 2001;22:392–8.
8. Evans J, Beingnessner D, Agel J, Benirschke SK. Minifragment plate fixation of high-energy navicular body fractures. Foot Ankle Int. 2011;32:485–92.
9. Schildhauer TA, Nork SE, Sangeorzan BJ. Temporary bridge plating of the medial column in severe midfoot injuries. J Orthop Trauma. 2003;17:513–20.

Chapter 14
Lisfranc Fracture/Dislocation Treated with Primary Arthrodesis

Clayton C. Bettin, Florian Nickisch, and Edward A. Perez

Case Presentation

A 66-year-old female presented to the outpatient clinic 4 days after a high-energy motor vehicle accident for evaluation of right-foot pain. She was a restrained driver who collided with a vehicle in front of her and had immediate pain and inability to bear weight on the right foot. She was initially evaluated at an outside hospital where she was informed that she dislocated her second metatarsophalangeal joint. A reduction was performed at the outside hospital, the right foot was splinted, and the patient was encouraged

C.C. Bettin, M.D. • E.A. Perez, M.D. (✉)
Department of Orthopaedic Surgery, University of Tennessee—Campbell Clinic, Memphis, TN 38104, USA
e-mail: perezmemphis@gmail.com

F. Nickisch, M.D.
Department of Orthopaedic Surgery, University of Utah School of Medicine, Salt Lake City, UT 84108, USA

N.C. Tejwani (ed.), *Fractures of the Foot and Ankle*,
DOI 10.1007/978-3-319-60456-5_14,

to follow up with a local podiatrist. The patient was evaluated 1 day prior to presentation by the podiatrist who recommended urgent surgical intervention for multiple fractures in the right foot. The patient presented to the orthopedic foot and ankle clinic for a second opinion. She has no prior injury to this foot until 4 days ago and no history of chronic foot pain. She has a history of controlled hypertension, depression, and hypothyroidism for which she takes appropriate medications. The patient is employed as a dental hygienist and denies tobacco, alcohol, or recreational drug use. She lives at home with her husband. She has been in overall good health until 4 days ago.

Physical examination of the patient shows her to have appropriate mood and affect. She has palpable pulses at regular rate and rhythm in all extremities and non-labored respirations. She has full range of motion of her neck without any tenderness to palpation. Her right foot shows significant swelling although her compartments are soft and compressible. There is ecchymosis extending plantarly from the toes to the heel. Her sensation is symmetric to her uninvolved extremity. She has significant tenderness to palpation in the midfoot as well as at the second metatarsophalangeal joint. There is no pain noted at her ankle, hindfoot, or base of the fifth metatarsal. Her second toe appears to be located clinically. She is able to dorsiflex and plantarflex her ankle and toes as well as invert and evert her hindfoot normally.

Injury Films

Non-weight bearing films were obtained in clinic secondary to the patient being unable to bear weight on the foot due to pain and are shown in Fig. 14.1. Interpretation of the

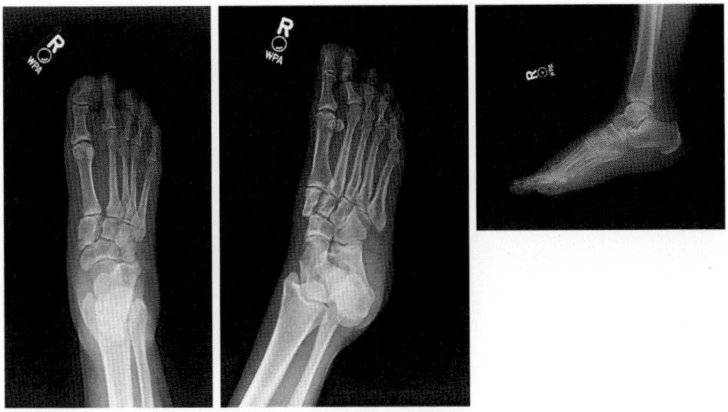

FIGURE 14.1 Injury AP, oblique, and lateral radiographs

radiographs shows widening of the first intermetatarsal space as well as between the medial and middle cuneiform. On the AP view, a line drawn from the medial navicular to the medial cuneiform and extended distally (Mills line) does not intersect the first metatarsal. There is an incongruous articulation between the navicular and medial cuneiform indicative of a longitudinal Lisfranc fracture dislocation with dislocation of the intercuneiform and naviculocuneiform joints. An avulsion-type fracture of the proximal medial pole of the medial cuneiform is apparent. The second MTP is reduced with slight varus angulation compared to the other MTP joints.

A CT scan was obtained to further evaluate the bony anatomy and is shown in Fig. 14.2. The fracture of the medial cuneiform is visualized, as is the shortening and dorsomedial translation of the naviculocuneiform joint consistent with a longitudinal Lisfranc injury pattern. Varus angulation of the second metatarsophalangeal joint is demonstrated.

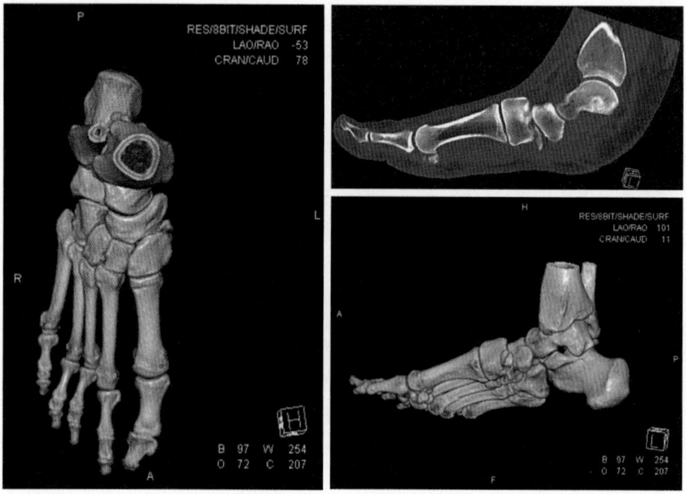

FIGURE 14.2 CT scan right foot

Treatment and Timing of Surgery

The patient was placed into a well-padded short leg splint. A long discussion was held with her regarding treatment options ranging from conservative to surgical. Due to the demonstrated instability at multiple joints, recommendation of surgical intervention with open reduction and internal fixation versus arthrodesis was given with determination of procedure based on assessment of cartilage intraoperatively. Risks of neurovascular injury, infection, persistent pain, and irritating hardware were discussed in detail and the patient signed informed consent for the procedure. Surgery was scheduled for 1 week later (12 days post-injury) to allow time for her soft-tissue swelling to resolve.

Surgical Technique

Position

After marking the surgical site and induction of general anesthesia with a popliteal block for postoperative pain control, the patient was positioned supine on the operating table with the feet at the edge of the bed. A right-thigh tourniquet was applied, intravenous antibiotics were given, and the extremity was prepped and draped in the standard surgical fashion. A time-out was taken to identify the correct patient, operative site, and other items per protocol. The limb was exsanguinated with an Esmarch and the tourniquet was insufflated to 275 mmHg.

Approach

An approximately 10 cm incision was made on the dorsum of the right foot and care was taken to protect the crossing branches of the superficial peroneal nerve. The interval between the extensor hallucis brevis and longus was identified and the brevis, along with the neurovascular bundle, was mobilized laterally with the longus taken medially. Significant disruption of the deep capsular structures was noted and hematoma was evacuated. Instability of the entire medial ray was visualized with disruption of the first intermetatarsal space, intercuneiform, and naviculocuneiform joints along with cartilaginous injury in the same. The first and second tarsometatarsal articulations were stable. The fracture of the proximal medial pole of the medial cuneiform was identified, found to be multifragmentary, and excised. Given the amount of instability, cartilage injury, and patient's age, the decision was made to proceed with arthrodesis of the intercuneiform, medial, and middle naviculocuneiform joints. Residual cartilage on the proximal and medial aspect of the medial cuneiform, lateral and proximal aspect of the middle cuneiform, and distal aspect of the medial and middle facets of the navicular was removed with a ¼" curved osteotomy and small curettes. A small lamina spreader and K-wire distractor were utilized as well to create enough distraction to ensure complete removal of cartilage from the plantar aspects of these joints. The subchondral bone of these articulations was then perforated using a water-cooled 2.0 mm drill bit. A 3 cm incision was made over Gerdy's tubercle on the right proximal tibia and dissection was carried down through the fascia onto the tubercle. The lateral wall was perforated by hand using a 6.5 mm drill guide and cancellous bone graft was removed using a large pituitary rongeur. The graft was morselized and packed into the interstices of the medial and middle naviculocuneiform, intercuneiform joints, and first intermetatarsal space.

Fracture Reduction and Fixation

Figure 14.3 shows the disruption of the medial ray as identified in the procedure, as well as provisional reduction obtained using a shoulder hook with an adduction and internal rotation maneuver to the medial ray. Attention should be paid to the restoration of Mills line (a line from the medial navicular to the medial cuneiform extended distally) as it now intersects the first metatarsal. The provisional reduction was held temporarily with 1.6 mm K-wires. An external compression device was utilized with appropriate wires to provide controlled compression of the medial ray. A medial incision was made just proximal to the navicular tuberosity and a 3.5 mm position screw was placed from the navicular into the medial cuneiform. Through the same medial incision, another 3.5 mm screw was placed from the navicular into the middle cuneiform. A clamp was placed across the first intermetatarsal space to compress the base of the second

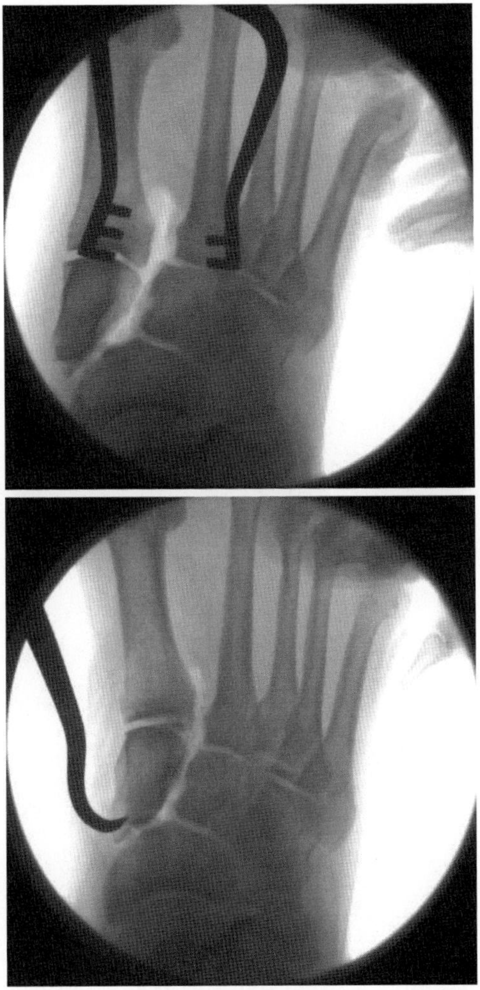

FIGURE 14.3 Provisional reduction

metatarsal to the medial cuneiform and a 3.5 mm position screw was placed through a stab incision medial to the cuneiform into the base of the second metatarsal. Retrograde 3.5 mm position screws were placed from the medial

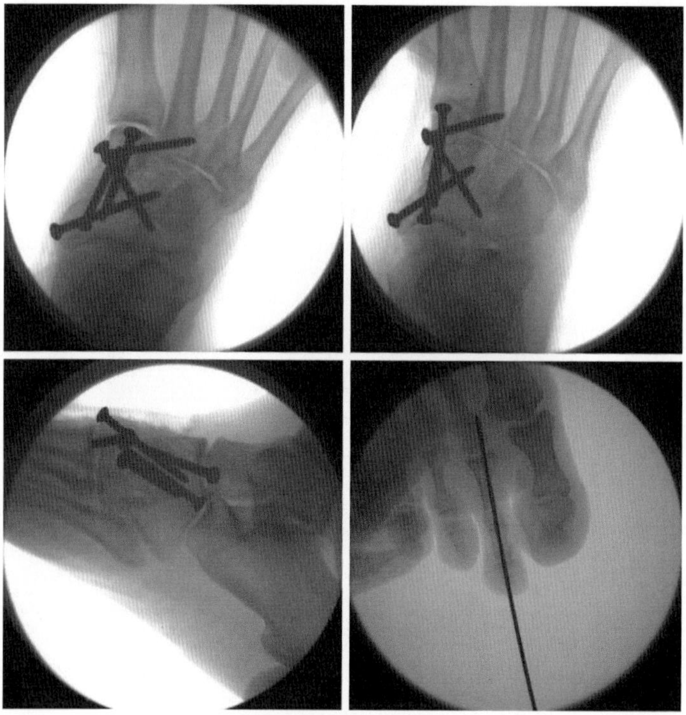

FIGURE 14.4 Final fluoroscopic images

cuneiform into the navicular as well as across the middle cuneiform and into the navicular. A 4-0 burr was used to create dorsal troughs in the navicular and medial/middle cuneiforms for additional strain-relieving bone graft to be packed into the interstices. The stability was tested and found to be excellent. The second MTP joint was held in a concentrically reduced position and a 1.6 mm K-wire was placed percutaneously retrograde from the tip of the toe, across the DIP, PIP, and MTP joints. Reduction and hardware position were checked fluoroscopically in multiple planes as shown in Fig. 14.4. All wounds were copiously irrigated and closed in a layered fashion. Sterile dressings were applied and a well-padded below-knee splint was applied.

Postoperative Plan

The patient returned at 2 weeks after surgery for wound inspection and suture removal. No wound complications were encountered. She was placed into a tall boot that was worn at all times other than when bathing for four additional weeks with strict nonweight-bearing precautions for the first 8 weeks after surgery. At 6 weeks boot removal for range of motion was allowed and the K-wire across the second MTP joint was removed. Progressive weight bearing began at 8 weeks after surgery.

Outcome

Radiographs were obtained at 6 weeks, 3 months, and 6 months post-op as shown in Figs. 14.5–14.7. A solid arthrodesis was obtained and at latest follow-up the patient had minimal pain and no limitations to her activities.

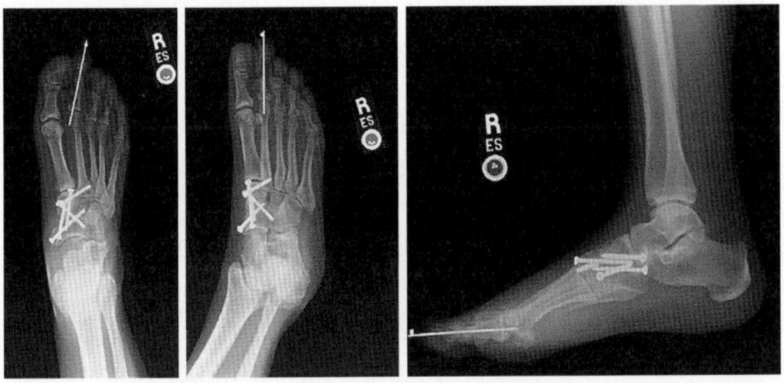

FIGURE 14.5 AP, oblique, and lateral radiographs 6 weeks post-op

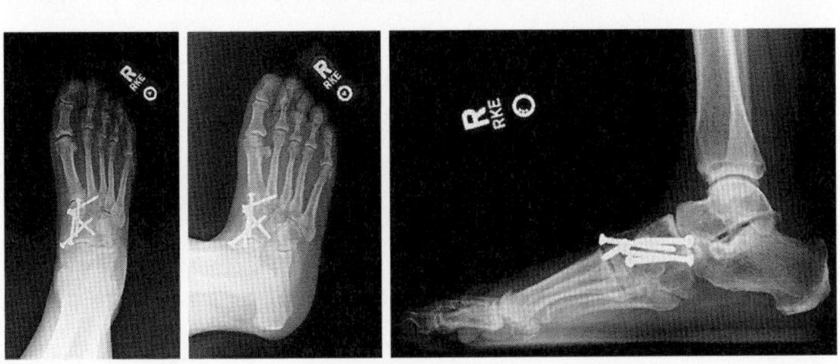

FIGURE 14.6 AP, oblique, and lateral radiographs 3 months post-op

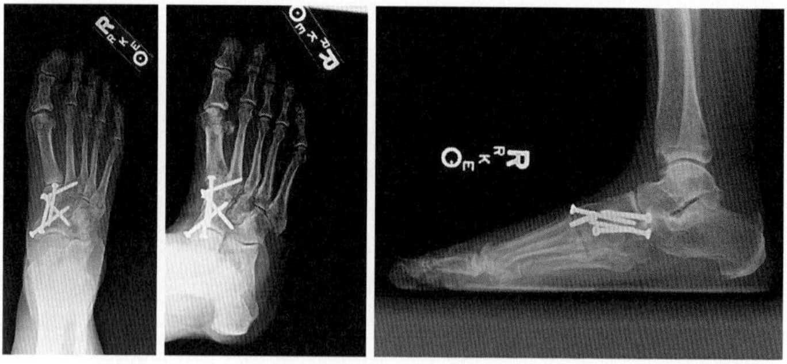

FIGURE 14.7 AP, oblique, and lateral radiographs 6 months post-op

Salient Points/Pearls

- A line drawn tangential to the medial navicular and cuneiform and extended distally should normally intersect the first metatarsal. This line is useful in detecting subtle Lisfranc injuries as well as in evaluating reduction during surgery [1].
- Both ORIF and arthrodesis are described as treatment for acute Lisfranc injuries. There is debate as to which is superior [2, 3]. Supporters of arthrodesis point out that there is poor potential for healing of the Lisfranc ligament back to bone with ORIF leading to later degenerative changes that may require arthrodesis. Many cases treated without arthrodesis undergo a second operation for planned hardware removal [4].
- Several studies have compared arthrodesis to ORIF, with arthrodesis having been shown to have a lower reoperation rate, similar patient outcomes, and similar rates of anatomic alignment obtained [4–8].
- Assessment of instability of midfoot joints should be made during surgery. All joints that demonstrate instability should be incorporated into the arthrodesis. Leaving an unstable joint will increase the likelihood of adjacent joint arthritis and need for future surgery.

- All articular cartilage from involved joints should be removed during arthrodesis procedure. Adequate joint distraction is imperative to visualize the most plantar aspects of the joint and assure that all cartilage is removed. Remaining plantar cartilage may increase the risk of nonunion.
- Cases of delayed diagnosis of a Lisfranc injury with degenerative changes of the articular surfaces should be treated with arthrodesis [9, 10].
- Most patients are able to return to their previous activities after arthrodesis for Lisfranc injuries however some patients do have limitations to activities after this injury which should be discussed preoperatively [11].

References

1. Coss HS, Manos RE, Buoncristiani A, Mills WJ. Abduction stress and AP weightbearing radiography of purely ligamentous injury in the tarsometatarsal joint. Foot Ankle Int. 1998;19(8):537–41.
2. Seybold JD, Coetzee JC. Lisfranc injuries: when to observe, fix, or fuse. Clin Sports Med. 2015;34:705–23.
3. Watson TS, Shurnas PS, Denker J. Treatment of Lisfranc joint injury: current concepts. J Am Acad Orthop Surg. 2010;18(12):718–28.
4. Ly TV, Coetzee JC. Treatment of primarily ligamentous Lisfranc joint injuries: primary arthrodesis compared with open reduction and internal fixation. A prospective, randomized study. J Bone Joint Surg. 2006;88(3):514–20.
5. Smith N, Stone C, Furey A. Does open reduction and internal fixation versus primary arthrodesis improve patient outcomes for Lisfranc trauma? A systematic review and meta-analysis. Clin Orthop Relat Res. 2016;474:1445–52.
6. Henning JA, Jones CB, Sietsema DL, Bohay DR, Anderson JG. Open reduction internal fixation versus primary arthrodesis for Lisfranc injuries: a prospective randomized study. Foot Ankle Int. 2009;30(10):913–22.
7. Reinhardt KR, LS O, Schottel P, Roberts MM, Levine D. Treatment of Lisfranc fracture-dislocations with primary partial arthrodesis. Foot Ankle Int. 2012;33(11):50–6.

8. Sheibani-Rad S, Coetzee JC, Giveans MR, Digiovanni C. Arthrodesis versus ORIF for Lisfranc fractures. Orthopedics. 2012;35(6):e868–73.
9. Aronow MS. Treatment of the missed Lisfranc injury. Foot Ankle Clin N Am. 2006;11:127–42.
10. Dubois-Ferriere V, Lubbeke A, Chowdhary A, Stern R, Dominguez D, Assal M. Clinical outcomes and development of symptomatic osteoarthritis 2 to 24 years after surgical treatment of tarsometatarsal joint complex injuries. J Bone Joint Surg. 2016;98:713–20.
11. MacMahon A, Kim P, Levine DS, Burket J, Roberts MM, Drakos MC, Deland JT, Elliott AJ, Ellis SJ. Return to sports and physical activities after primary partial arthrodesis for Lisfranc injuries in young patients. Foot Ankle Int. 2016;37(4):355–62.

Chapter 15
Lisfranc Fracture/Dislocation Treated with ORIF

Daniela Sanchez, Daniel Scott Horwitz, Amrut Borade, and Harish Kempegowda

Abbreviations

AP	Anteroposterior
ORIF	Open reduction and internal fixation
TMT	Tarsometatarsal

Case Presentation

A 31-year-old male patient presented to the office with pain in his left foot for 3 days secondary to an injury sustained while playing football. He was pushed from the back when his foot was in a plantar-flexed position, suffering from what appeared to be a hyperextension injury to the midfoot. The patient felt a crack/pop sensation followed by severe pain

D. Sanchez, M.D. • D.S. Horwitz, M.D. (✉)
A. Borade, M.B.B.S., M.S. • H. Kempegowda, M.B.B.S., M.S.
Department of Orthopaedics, Geisinger Health System,
100 N Academy Ave., Danville, PA 17821, USA
e-mail: dshorwitz@geisinger.edu

N.C. Tejwani (ed.), *Fractures of the Foot and Ankle*,
DOI 10.1007/978-3-319-60456-5_15,

and swelling. The patient was non-weight bearing in his left foot but the pain failed to subside for 3 days. On exam, even though there was no evident plantar ecchymosis which would be a sign highly suggestive of a Lisfranc injury, diffuse soft-tissue swelling was documented over the first and second metatarsal bases, and midfoot movements caused significant pain and discomfort. Movement of the ankle joint, fore foot, and hind foot was pain free. His neurovascular exam was normal without any open wounds over the foot, and no signs of compartment syndrome were noted.

Treatment Considerations and Planning

If a Lisfranc injury is suspected, one should obtain anteroposterior (AP), lateral, and oblique radiographs of the foot in order to evaluate congruency of the tarsometatarsal (TMT) complex [1]. The AP view is used to evaluate the first and second TMT joints, the oblique view will allow the evaluation of the alignment of the third and fourth TMT joints, and the lateral view of the foot will be useful for the assessment of dorsal and plantar dislocations of the Lisfranc joint [2]. A Lisfranc injury is diagnosed when the medial base of the second metatarsal is not lined up with medial aspect of the middle cuneiform on an AP view. A pathognomonic radiologic sign is the "*fleck sign*" [3] between the bases of the first and second metatarsals, which indicates an avulsion of the Lisfranc ligament from either the medial cuneiform or the base of the second metatarsal. For patients with a subtle lesion, a stress radiograph consisting of a weight-bearing AP X-ray of both feet may help make the diagnosis of a Lisfranc injury if there is an increased joint space between the first and second metatarsals with respect to the uninjured foot [4]. In order to perform an adequate stress test, the weight should be evenly distributed on both feet, which may be painful for the patient; therefore in some cases using local anesthesia before taking the radiographs may help improve the quality of the test [1]. CT scans are useful among patients with

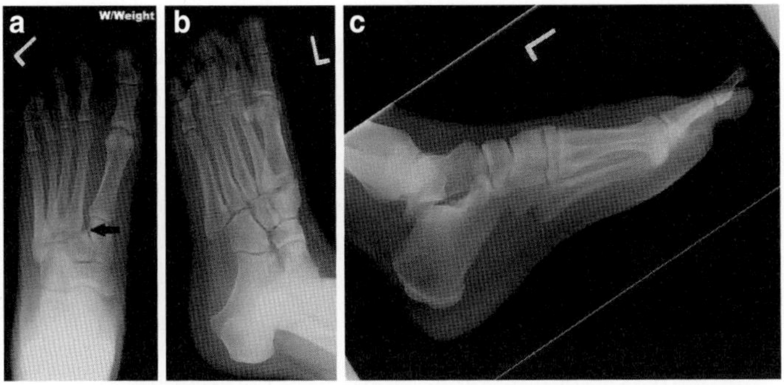

FIGURE 15.1 Radiographs of the patient's left foot taken 3 days after the injury. (**a**) Weight-bearing AP view showing >2 mm diastasis of the first intermetatarsal space and loss of alignment between the medial borders of the middle cuneiform and the base of the second metatarsal. The arrow is showing the *fleck sign*: an avulsion of the Lisfranc ligament from the base of the second metatarsal. (**b**) Oblique view shows congruent third and fourth TMT joints. (**c**) Lateral view showing no dorsal or plantar displacements

complex fractures who require a more accurate delineation of the fracture pattern. If there is no clear evidence of displacement in the X-rays but there is a suspicion of a Lisfranc injury then a MRI may help detect a sprain or rupture of the ligament.

In this case, the standard radiographs including AP, lateral, and oblique views of the left foot were obtained (Fig. 15.1). The AP radiograph revealed findings of 5.5 mm diastasis at the first inter-metatarsal space and a disturbed linear relation between the second metatarsal and the middle cuneiform, both findings consistent with the diagnosis of Lisfranc injury. The lateral three rays of the left foot appeared congruent on the oblique view and there was no evidence of vertical instability on the lateral view.

The first step in the management of any Lisfranc injury is to decide whether surgical fixation is needed. Anatomic reduction and internal fixation is the preferred option for injuries with a diastasis of more than 2 mm at the first metatarsal space [1, 5].

The different fixation options are screws, low profile plates, interosseous sutures, and K-wires, but, regardless of the implant used for fixation, the mainstay of treatment is to obtain an anatomic reduction of the Lisfranc joint, stabilizing the medial and middle columns of the foot while preserving motion of the lateral column [1, 5–7]. The advantages and limitations of various treatment modalities are as follows.

Screws: They remain the most popular treatment option, representing approximately 82% of the implants used for internal fixation of Lisfranc fractures [5]. Compared to fixation with Kirschner pins, small fragment fully threaded screws have better biomechanical features; they achieve superior stabilization and tolerate higher bearing forces without loss of reduction [7, 8]. On the other hand, they are transarticular implants with an inherent risk of causing thermal injury to cartilage possibly resulting in an increased risk of posttraumatic arthritis [9]. Another disadvantage of screws is the necessity for hardware removal. Although most authors suggest that screws should be removed between the third and sixth postoperative months, there is still no clear evidence regarding the indications for removal and when should this surgery be performed [1, 10].

Interosseous suture techniques: Open reduction and internal fixation (ORIF) using suture techniques have been recently developed trying to overcome the problem of damaging the articular surface with screws and possibly decreasing the incidence of posttraumatic arthritis. Studies have shown equivalent stability compared to screws, and suture systems do not require an additional procedure for hardware removal [11, 12]. Theoretically, suture techniques can be effectively used for fixation because they mimic the Lisfranc ligament and can help maintain reduction, making them a suitable treatment option for athletes [2, 13, 14]. There is inadequate evidence to support a routine use of this technique over screws.

Plates: Low-profile plates have been utilized in the treatment of Lisfranc injuries; they are joint-spanning implants and therefore are less likely to cause damage to the articular surface, and they are removed only if the patient becomes symptomatic [1]. The surgical approach and exposure are wider with respect to the approach needed for screws and this can compromise blood supply and soft tissues, potentially affecting bone healing [15]. Although to date there are no clear indications for their use, plates are helpful for ORIF of comminuted fractures [1]. The stability achieved with plates is similar to the stability obtained when using trans-articular screws and loss of reduction with weight-bearing forces is comparable to screws [16, 17].

Based on these factors, the decision was made to perform ORIF with screws.

Intraoperative Tips and Tricks for Reduction and Fixation

The procedure was performed with the patient in a supine position with his knee flexed and using a triangular support in order to allow a plantigrade position of the foot. A dorsal longitudinal incision over the first TMT joint space between the extensor hallucis longus and the extensor hallucis brevis tendons was made. The neurovascular bundle was carefully preserved while exposing the first intermetatarsal space. Under direct visualization, the first TMT joint was tested and found to be unstable, so the first ray was stabilized with an axial screw from the metatarsal to the medial cuneiform and a pointed reduction clamp was then placed across the medial cuneiform to the second metatarsal base to reduce the Lisfranc complex. The Lisfranc screw was placed from the medial aspect of the medial cuneiform to the second metatarsal base and the second metatarsal was additionally stabilized with a screw from the base to the middle cuneiform. Intraoperatively, the third metatarsal was stressed and found to be unstable; hence a screw was placed across the third TMT joint. The lateral column was stable when tested intraoperatively; therefore no further fixation was required. Finally, the quality of the reduction was confirmed clinically and radiographically (Fig. 15.2).

In cases where the joints in the lateral column are found to be unstable, attempts for close reduction and percutaneous fixation can be done. If reduction cannot be maintained,

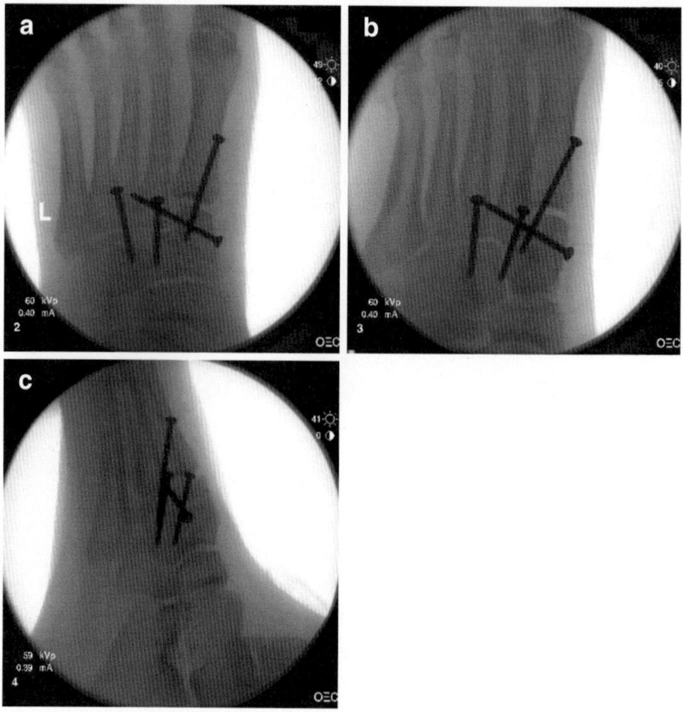

FIGURE 15.2 Fluoroscopic images of the final reduction and fixation of the Lisfranc injury. (**a**) AP view showing fixation with a Lisfranc screw. Note that the medial borders of the second metatarsal and the middle cuneiform are aligned. The first and second metatarsals are fixed to the medial and middle cuneiforms, respectively, using fully threaded screws. (**b**) Oblique view shows the third metatarsal fixed to the lateral cuneiform and congruent fourth and fifth TMT joints. (**c**) No vertical instability documented on the lateral view

or is difficult to achieve by these means, open reduction is required. A dorsal longitudinal incision over the fourth intermetatarsal space will allow access to the third and fourth TMT joints and reduction under direct visualization can be performed. Flexible fixation with Kirschner wires will help maintain reduction without completely restricting motion of the lateral column and they are typically removed after 6 weeks [1, 10].

Key Points/Pearls

- Make longitudinal incisions to address the affected joints: A dorsomedial approach will give access to the first and second TMT joints and a dorsolateral approach will give access to the TMT in the lateral column. *Beware:* Protect skin flaps to avoid necrosis [10].
- If anatomic reduction can't be obtained look for soft-tissue interposition (tibialis anterior tendon) [1, 18].
- The sequence of reduction of Lisfranc fractures should go from proximal to distal and from medial to lateral, reducing and temporarily fixing the medial column first, following reduction of the middle and lateral columns [10, 18].
- Anatomic reduction and rigid fixation of the medial and middle columns + flexible fixation (pins) of the lateral column if needed [19].
- The Lisfranc screw can be placed from the base of the second metatarsal towards the medial cuneiform as the target is bigger [15].
- Avoid using lag or partially threaded screws because they can increase stress across the articular surface [2].
- Always evaluate the quality and stability of the fixation.

Postoperative Protocols and Follow-Up

The patient was kept nonweight bearing in a splint during the first 6 weeks and was encouraged to slowly advance to full weight bearing over the next 4–6 weeks. By the end of 12 weeks the patient was full weight bearing in his regular shoes.

Controversy remains regarding screw removal and the timing of the procedure. Although the patient did not develop hardware-related symptoms, when the risks and benefits of hardware removal were explained, he opted for screw removal and the surgery was performed after 5 months. At 1-year follow-up, the patient reported no complaints and did not have difficulty in carrying out his regular activities. Radiographs obtained revealed a well-aligned foot with well-maintained reduction of the Lisfranc joint and there were no degenerative changes (Fig. 15.3).

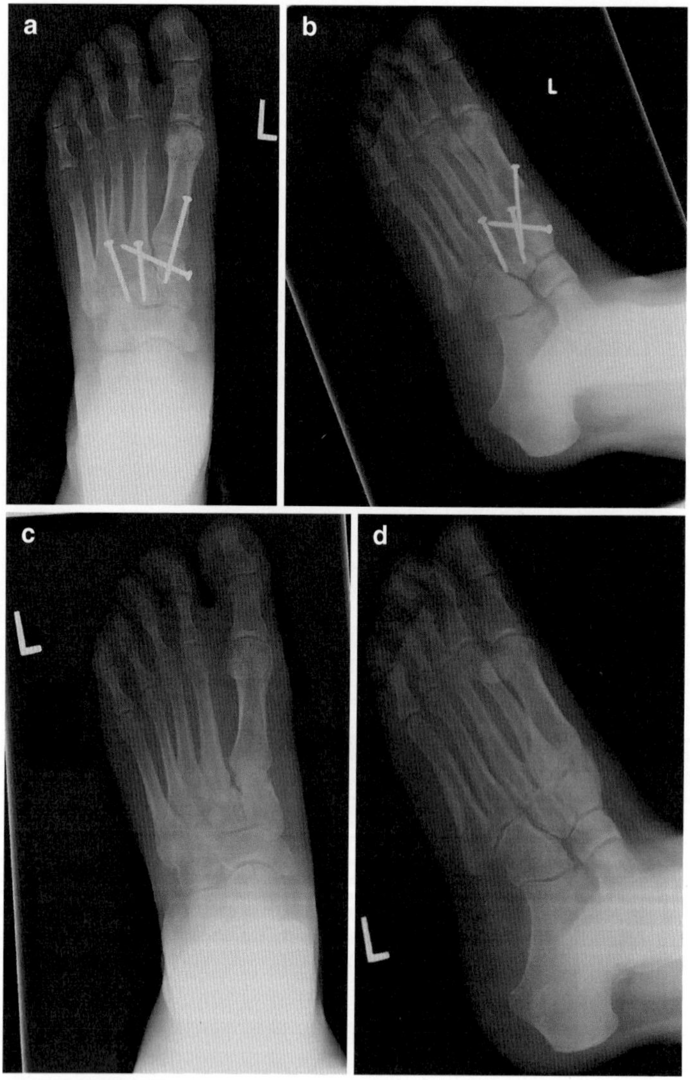

FIGURE 15.3 Follow-up X-rays at 3 months and 1 year postoperative. (**a**) and (**b**) AP and oblique views at the third postoperative month showing that the reduction is maintained and no implant failure. (**c**) and (**d**) AP and oblique views at 1-year follow-up. Screws have been removed and reduction of Lisfranc joint has been maintained

Another Mode of Treatment

Here we have a similar clinical scenario of a pure ligamentous Lisfranc injury of the right foot of a male adult sustained while he was practicing football. Additional to the initial set of X-rays, a stress test was performed and demonstrated instability of the Lisfranc complex (Fig. 15.4).

As joint instability was documented, the decision to proceed with surgical treatment was made and the patient underwent ORIF with interosseous sutures. In this case the reduction of the Lisfranc complex was maintained using a tenaculum clamp while a guide wire was placed from the medial cuneiform to the base of the second metatarsal in a percutaneous fashion. After confirmation of the position of

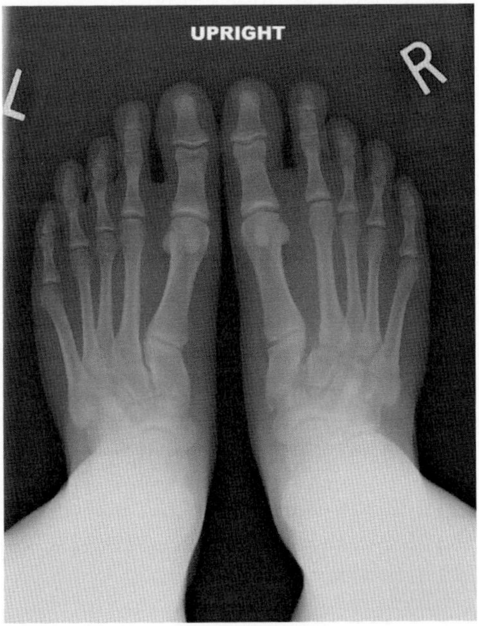

FIGURE 15.4 Shows full weight-bearing AP views of both feet (stress test). The first intermetatarsal joint space is >1 mm wider with respect to the left foot

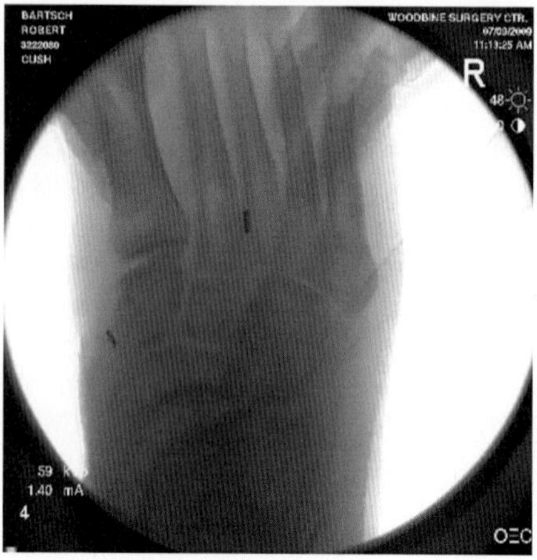

FIGURE 15.5 Fluoroscopic AP view of the reduced Lisfranc complex and its fixation using and interosseous suture

the guide wire using biplanar fluoroscopy, a drill hole was made using a 2.7 mm drill bit to allow the passage of the tightrope needle. Subsequently, the needle was passed through the drill hole, an anchor was pulled through and engaged on the medial cortex of the medial cuneiform, and the button was tightened down at the base of the second metatarsal (Fig. 15.5). Finally, the stability of the reduction was checked under fluoroscopy and no instability of the TMT joints was evidenced.

During the follow-up period, the postoperative protocol was similar to the one described previously. At his last follow-up, the patient was asymptomatic and tolerated full weight bearing. The X-rays showed a reduced Lisfranc joint and no failure of fixation materials (Fig. 15.6).

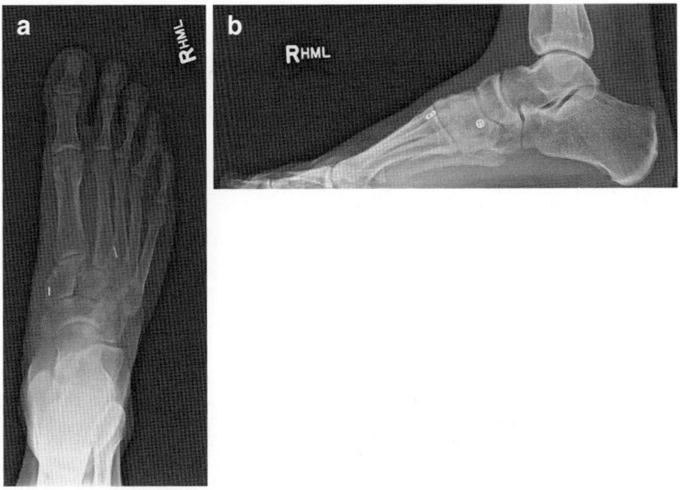

FIGURE 15.6 Follow-up X-rays at 3 months postoperative showing maintenance of reduction and no implant failure in both AP (**a**) and lateral views (**b**)

Outcomes

Although there are multiple short- and long-term complications (compartment syndrome, neurovascular injuries, flat foot deformity, and chronic instability), posttraumatic arthritis continues to be the most common problem after Lisfranc injuries [10]. The most important factors contributing to this are the extent of the initial injury and the quality of the reduction after ORIF. Regardless of which implants are used for internal fixation, an anatomic reduction is the main determinant for achieving good clinical outcomes [6]. Although approximately 50% of patients will have arthritic radiographic changes in the follow-up X-rays, not all patients are symptomatic, and only 7–8% require arthrodesis [5].

ORIF of severe fracture dislocations are associated with less pain and less stiffness compared to primary arthrodesis [10, 15]. As discussed, anatomic and stable ORIF can be achieved using either screws or interosseous sutures; however the advantages and limitations of these implants must be considered in order to choose the appropriate implant for each individual patient.

Although current evidence suggests that better clinical outcomes are obtained when primary arthrodesis is performed in patients with purely ligamentous injuries [6, 10] the evidence comparing the use of arthrodesis vs. ORIF with interosseous sutures for treating this type of injury remains scarce. Despite a lack of strong evidence, fixation using interosseous sutures may be advantageous, especially in athletes as it allows early weight bearing, doesn't require hardware removal, and preserves midfoot mobility [2].

References

1. Watson TS, Shurnas PS, Denker J. Treatment of lisfranc joint injury: current concepts. J Am Acad Orthop Surg. 2010;18:718–28.
2. Seybold JD, Coetzee CJ. Lisfranc injuries when to observe, fix, or fuse. Clin Sports Med. 2015;34(4):705–23. doi:10.1016/j.csm.2015.06.006.
3. Myerson M, Fisher R, Burgess A, Kenzora JE. Fracture dislocations of the oetatarsal joints: end results correlated with pathology and treatment. Foot Ankle. 1986;6(5):225–42.
4. Nunley JA, Vertullo CJ. Classification, investigation and management of midfoot sprains. Am J Sports Med. 2002;30:871–8.
5. Stavlas P, Roberts CS, Xypnitos FN, Giannoudis PV. The role of reduction and internal fixation of Lisfranc fracture – dislocations: a systematic review of the literature. Int Orthop. 2010;34:1083–91.
6. Mulier T, Haan de J, Vriesendorp P, Reynders P. The treatment of lisfranc injuries: review of current literature. Eur J Trauma Emerg Surg. 2010;36:206–16.
7. Zgonis T, Roukis TS, Polyzois VD. Lisfranc fracture-dislocations: current treatment and new surgical approaches. Clin Podiatr Med Surg. 2006;23:303–22.

8. Lee CA, Birkedal JP, Dickerson EA, Vieta PA, Webb LX, Teasdall RD. Stabilization of Lisfranc joint injuries: a biomechanical study. Foot Ankle Int. 2004;25(5):365–70.
9. Eleftheriou KI, Rossenfeld PF, Calder JDF. Lisfranc injuries: an update. Knee Surg Sports Traumatol Arthrosc. 2013;21:1434–46.
10. Welck MJ, Zinchenko R, Rudge B. Lisfranc injuries. Injury. 2015;46(4):536–41. doi:10.1016/j.injury.2014.11.026.
11. Panchbhavi VK, Vallurupalli S, Yang J, Andersen CR. Screw fixation compared with suture-button fixation of isolated lisfranc injuries. J Bone Joint Surg Am. 2009;91(5):1143–8.
12. Pelt CE, Bachus KN, Vance RE, Beals TC. A biomechanical analysis of a tensioned suture device in the fixation of the ligamentous lisfranc injury. Foot Ankle Int. 2011;32(4):422–31.
13. Cottom JM, Hyer CF, Berlet GC. Treatment of lisfranc fracture dislocations with an interosseous suture botton technique: a review of 3 cases. J Foot Ankle Surg. 2008;47(3):250–8.
14. Brin YS, Nyska M, Kish B. Lisfranc injury repair with the tightrope device: a short-term case series. Foot Ankle Int. 2010;31(7):624–7.
15. Panchbhavi VK. Current operative techniques in lisfranc injury. Oper Tech Orthop. 2008;18:239–46. doi:10.1053/j.oto.2009.02.003.
16. Alberta FG, Aronow MS, Ma B, Diaz-Doran V, Sullivan RS, Adams DJ. Ligamentous Lisfranc joint injuries: a biomechanical comparison of dorsal plate and transarticula screw fixation. Foot Ankle Int. 2005;26(6):462–73.
17. Stern RE, Assal M. Dorsal multiple plating without routine transarticular screws for fixation of lisfranc injury. Orthopedics. 2014;37(12):815–9.
18. Benirschle SK, Meinberg E, Anderson SA, Jones CB, Cole PA. IFractures and dislocations of the midfoot: lisfranc and chopart injuries. J Bone Joint Surg Br. 2012;94-A:1325–37.
19. Mak JCS, Cameron ID, March LM. Evidence-based guidelines for the management of hip fractures in older persons: an update. Med J Aust. 2010;192(1):37–41.

Chapter 16
Fifth Metatarsal Fracture Treated with Intramedullary Screw Fixation

Kathryn O'Connor

Case Presentation

A 51-year-old, morbidly obese male presented to the office 5 days after injuring his right foot. He reported that earlier in the week he was walking across the street and, when he stepped off the curb, felt a "pop" on the outside of the foot. He had persistent pain for 2–3 days and ultimately went to the emergency room where he was found to have a fracture at the base of the fifth metatarsal. He denied any prodromal symptoms, and had no history of falls or trauma to the foot.

K. O'Connor, M.D., M.S.P.T.
Department of Orthopaedics, University of Pennsylvania, Philadelphia, PA 19104, USA
e-mail: Kathryn.O'connor@uphs.upenn.edu

N.C. Tejwani (ed.), *Fractures of the Foot and Ankle*,
DOI 10.1007/978-3-319-60456-5_16,

On examination, he had increased prominence on the base of the fifth metatarsal in standing, a flexible varus position of his heel, and adduction of his forefoot in standing. In addition, he had weakness in his peroneals and, when walking, made initial contact on the lateral border of his foot.

Injury Films

Non-weight bearing imaging of the foot shows a nondisplaced fracture of the proximal aspect of the fifth metatarsal. The fracture was located in "zone 2" of the fifth metatarsal, was transverse, and at the level of the 4/5 metatarsal articulation. This is all consistent with a "Jones" fracture. His repeat images more clearly show the fracture line (Fig. 16.1).

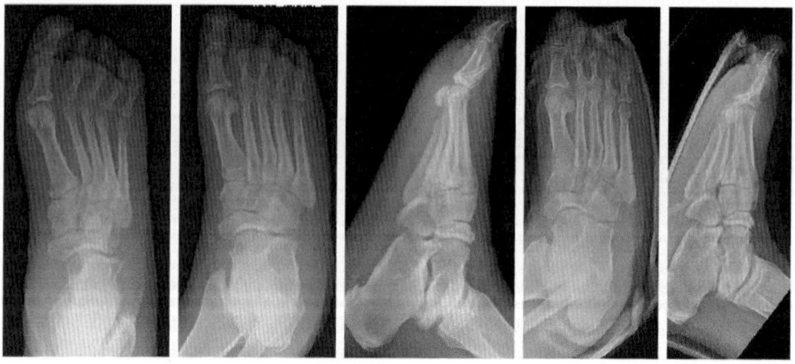

Figure 16.1 Three non-weight bearing images of the foot initial images, and images 2 days later

Treatment and Timing of Surgery

While most literature focuses on fractures of the fifth metatarsal in the athlete, this case reviews other scenarios where fixation may be beneficial to promote healing. Current recommendations are for surgical fixation in patients who are actively engaged in high level athletics so as to enable a faster return to training [1, 2]. In the remainder of the population, there is controversy over whether surgical fixation is necessary or whether fractures can best be managed non-weight bearing in a cast. Nonunion rates in patients treated nonoperatively have been reported in a wide range, but average in the area of 15–20%, compared to 5% in operative fixation [1, 3]. Some evidence indicates that hindfoot varus may be a predisposing factor to Jones fractures and nonunions [3].

In this patient we discussed operative and nonoperative treatment, and began with a trial to see if he would be able to maintain non-weight bearing. Unfortunately, due to his size he was unable to adequately maintain non-weight bearing, and the decision was made to proceed with fixation. This was deemed the best chance of healing since, in this scenario, his mechanism was consistent with a stress fracture and we were unable to remove the inciting stresses.

Surgical Tact

Position

The patient can be positioned supine or side lying with the affected side up. The author's preference is for side lying as it

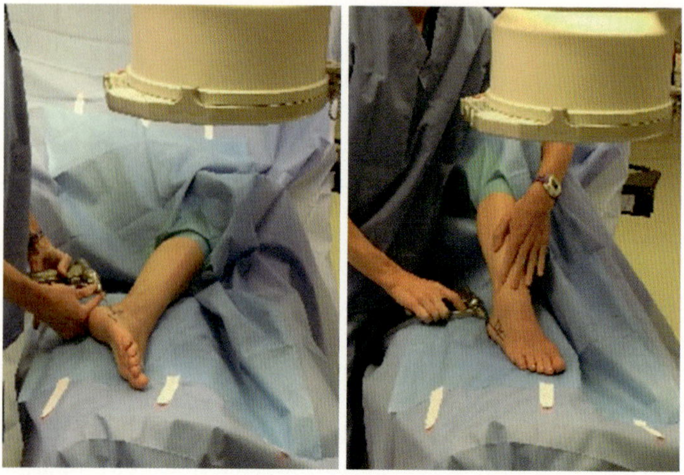

FIGURE 16.2 Setup with the patient sidelying. AP and lateral imaging can be done with very little manipulation of the leg

places the surgeon in a more advantageous position to place the guidewire. In the lateral position you are able to advance the guidewire without needing assistance to support or hold the leg; this is especially helpful if operating alone. The non-operative leg is positioned anteriorly, and the surgical leg is positioned on a stack of towels or blankets to make a supportive working surface. A large or small C-Arm can be used to image the foot, but it is this surgeon's preference to use the large C-Arm to prevent moving the foot while trying to obtain the starting point (Fig. 16.2).

Approach

Fluoroscopy is used to identify the level of the incision by obtaining a lateral X-ray and placing the incision in line with the canal of the fifth metatarsal (Fig. 16.3). The incision is approximately 2 cm in length starting 1–2 cm proximal to the base of the fifth metatarsal. Once through the skin, careful

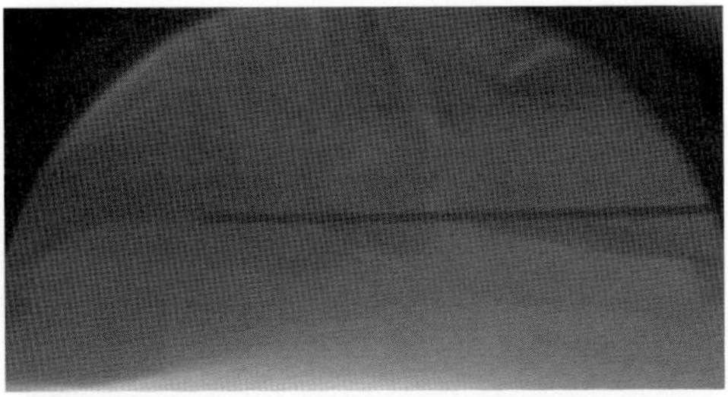

FIGURE 16.3 Lateral Images to help determine level of incision

dissection down to the base of the metatarsal is performed to be sure that crossing branches of the sural or superficial peroneal nerve are not injured. In addition, this allows spreading and protection of the peroneal tendons. Throughout the case, tissue protectors should be used to protect these structures during drilling and tapping.

Reduction and Fixation

Much like all other intramedullary devices, the critical step of the procedure is getting the appropriate starting point. In the fifth metatarsal this is frequently described as the "high and inside" position (Fig. 16.4) [4]. On AP, lateral, and oblique images there needs to be a straight line down the center of the canal with the guidewire. Using fluoroscopy, the guidewire is carefully advanced to a central place within the canal. The shape of the fifth metatarsal is generally over 4 mm in diameter with a slight curve in the distal half of the bone. This prevents placing the guidewire along the length of the intramedullary canal. It is important not to over-advance the guidewire, tap or drill, and perforate distal cortex creating a distal stress riser.

The fracture line is generally found approximately 20 mm from the base of the bone, and it is imperative that the guidewire is advanced far enough to have the screw threads cross this site [5]. Once the guidewire is placed, an over-drill and tap are used to prepare the canal (Fig. 16.5). A solid, partially

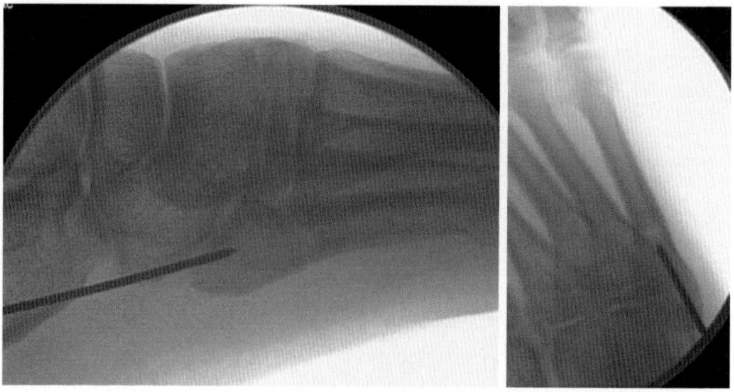

FIGURE 16.4 Obtaining starting point

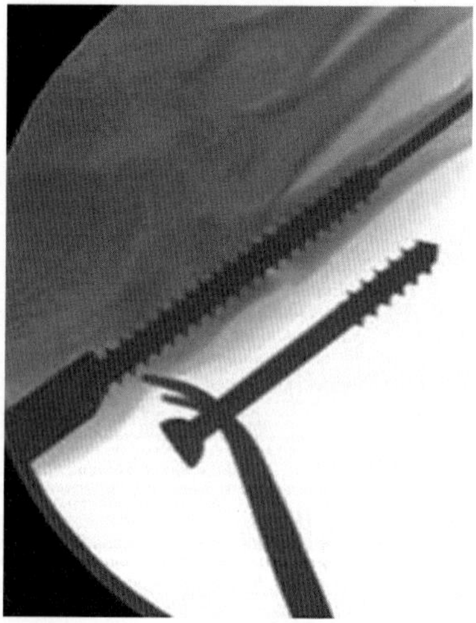

FIGURE 16.5 Measuring screw to check that threads cross the fracture site while tapping the canal

threaded screw provides the greatest stiffness and allows for compression of the fracture site. This has become the current standard fixation method [2, 5]. When choosing screw length, it is important that all of the threads cross the facture site. However, the screw should not be too long and distract the fracture site if it engages distally [4]. The screw is advanced until it gets adequate purchase (Figs. 16.6).

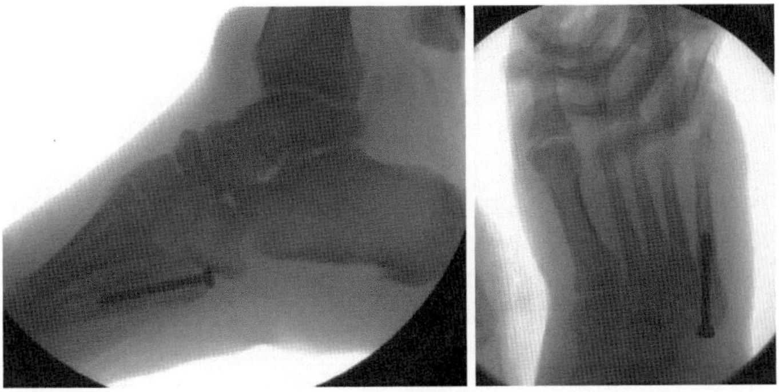

FIGURE 16.6 Immediate postoperative images

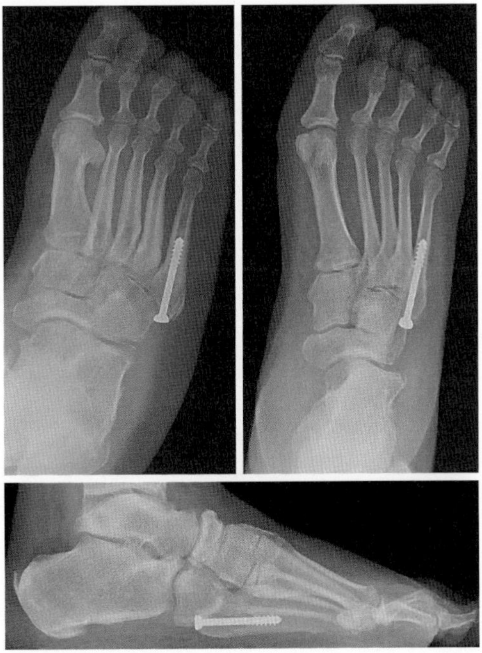

FIGURE 16.7 Final follow-up image-sat 6 months postoperative

Postoperative Plan

Immediately postoperatively, the patient is placed into a plaster splint and made non-weight bearing. At the 2-week postoperative appointment, sutures are removed. Due to this particular patient's obesity and difficulty maintaining NWB, he was maintained in a cast for 6 weeks and attempted to be NWB as best as he could manage, primarily heel weight bearing. He was then transitioned to a walker boot to begin weight bearing as tolerated at 6 weeks post-op. A custom ankle foot orthotic was made to help hold his heel in a neutral alignment and thereby prevent heel strike on the outside border of the foot. The patient transitioned into this at the 10-week mark once it was fabricated.

Additionally, since this patient's vitamin D levels were subphysiologic, he was supplemented with a 12-week course of 50,000 units.

Postoperatively this patient's case was handled more conservatively than normally due his the obesity. For most patients, as described in many protocols, weight bearing as tolerated can begin as early as 2–4 weeks with transition into a boot at that time [2, 4].

Outcome

The patient went on to full cortical bridging on X-rays at approximately 3 months (Fig. 16.7). He had no pain at his fracture site. He continues to use the custom ankle brace for ambulation to help prevent repeat stress to the lateral border of the foot.

Salient Points/Pearls

- Optimizing patients with vitamin D may be beneficial to aid in healing and preventing nonunion.
- Starting point of guidewire is the critical step in the procedure; it is important to make sure this is in exact location.

- If there is concern about distraction at the fracture site, then trying a shorter screw may help to reduce the risk of the screw distracting the site before it has gotten adequate purchase in the medullary canal.
- A shorter, wider screw is preferable to a longer, thinner screw, so long as all threads cross the fracture site and provide compression [4].
- Clamping the fracture may be possible using percutaneous incisions and a large pointed reduction clamp across the fracture if there are signs of distraction [6].
- For first time fracture fixation, there is no clear indication for use of augments such as bone marrow aspirate, or bone grafting. This may be indicated for cases of nonunion.
- In cases of nonunions, an examination of the patients' hindfoot alignment is necessary to determine if overall foot posture is contributing to excessive forces at the base of the fifth metatarsal. Occasionally, hindfoot osteotomies may be necessary to correct varus alignment [3, 4].

References

1. Bishop J, et al. Operative versus nonoperative treatment of jones fractures: a decision analysis model. Am J Orthop. 2016;45(2):E69–76.
2. Lareau C, et al. Return to play in national football league players after operative jones fracture treatment. Foot Ankle Int. 2016;37(1):8–16.
3. Rakin S, et al. The association of varus hindfoot and fracture of the fifth metatarsal metaphyseal-diaphyseal junction: the Jones fracture. Am J Sports Med. 2008;36(7):1367–72.
4. Nunley J. Jones fracture technique. Tech Foot Ankle Surg. 2002;1(2):131–7.
5. Ochenjele G. Radiographic study of the fifth metatarsal for optimal intramedullary screw fixation of jones fracture. Foot Ankle Int. 2015;36(3):293–301.
6. Tan E, et al. Use of percutaneous pointed reduction clamp before screw fixation to prevent gapping of a fifth metatarsal base fracture: a technique tip. J Foot Ankle Surg. 2016;55(1):151–6.

Chapter 17
Metatarsal Fractures Fixed with Plates or Wires

Megan Reilly and Saqib Rehman

History

A 28-year-old female presented to the trauma bay with bilateral foot and ankle pain after a fall from two stories in an apparent suicide attempt. Apart from substance abuse and suicidal ideation, she had no significant past medical history. On physical examination, she had right dorsal foot swelling, ecchymosis, and lateral foot abrasions, but her compartments were soft. She was able to dorsiflex and plantar flex the hallux and the ankle. She had normal sensation over the dorsum of the foot, the first web space, and the plantar aspect of the foot with a palpable dorsalis pedis pulse. In her right foot, she was found to have segmental second and third metatarsal fractures (Fig. 17.1a–c), a minimally displaced medial calcaneal fracture, and minimally displaced lateral and medial cuneiform fractures.

M. Reilly, M.D. • S. Rehman, M.D. (✉)
Department of Orthopaedic Surgery, Temple University, Philadelphia, PA, USA
e-mail: saqib.rehman@tuhs.temple.edu

N.C. Tejwani (ed.), *Fractures of the Foot and Ankle*,
DOI 10.1007/978-3-319-60456-5_17,

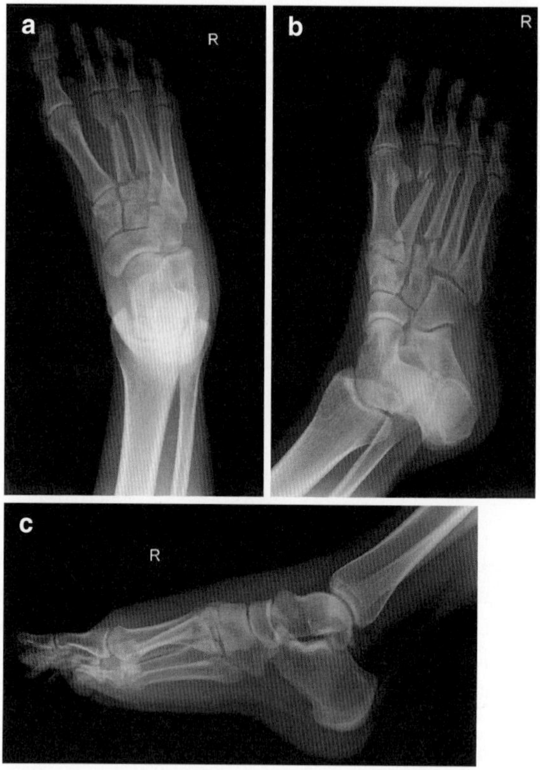

FIGURE 17.1 Right foot trauma bay radiographs after initial injury. (**a**) (AP), (**b**) (oblique), (**c**) (lateral). Segmental second and third metatarsal fractures with 100% transverse displacement of the distal fractures

Associated injuries included a left minimally displaced posterior inferior calcaneal fracture. She was splinted in a bulky padded posterior splint and elevated. Her vital signs remained stable during her hospitalization and diagnostic imaging of her chest, abdomen, and pelvis showed no additional injuries. Because of her edematous foot, she was unable to undergo immediate surgery, so she was instructed to keep it elevated within the splint. The concern was that the foot swelling could compromise her chances to have an adequately healing, or even closeable, wound. She was discharged to an inpatient psychiatric facility to address her immediate psychiatric needs.

Operative Planning

The patient presented at 5 weeks after injury; these blisters were healed. Radiographs of the right foot included an AP, lateral, and oblique view, which exhibited transverse fractures of the proximal and distal aspects of the right second and third metatarsals (Fig. 17.2a–c). Since her proximal metatarsal fractures had started to heal with minimal displacement, it was determined that only the distal fractures would be addressed in the operating room in order to correct the malalignment. Typically, proximal metatarsal fractures have bony support and little ligamentous disruption, which make

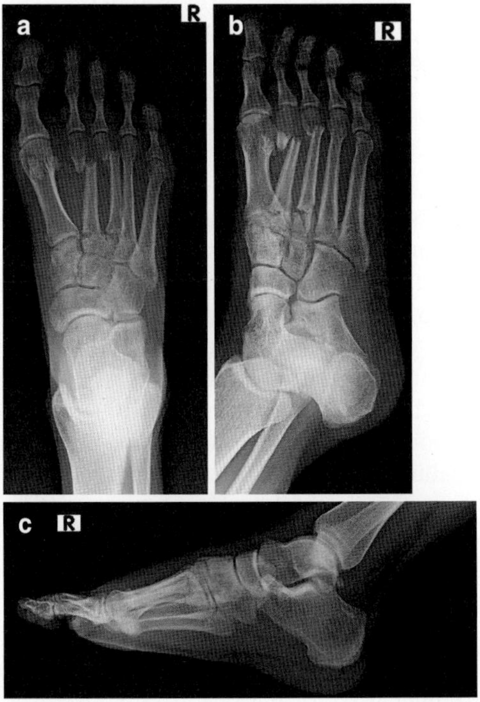

FIGURE 17.2 Right foot radiographs 5 weeks after initial injury. (**a**) (AP), (**b**) (oblique), (**c**) (lateral). Second and third metatarsal fractures as previously described, still with displaced distal fractures with evidence of interval callus formation

them stable and nondisplaced, and they respond well to non-operative treatment [1]. Because of the very distal nature of the third metatarsal fracture, it was determined that a plate would likely not get enough screw purchase for stable fixation—therefore the fracture would be pinned.

Indications for fixation of metatarsal shaft fractures vary—typically similar rules apply for all metatarsals except for the proximal fifth metatarsal fracture. Generally, displacement can be tolerated in the transverse plan, but sagittal plane displacement can lead to prominent metatarsal heads during weight bearing. The most consistent recommendations for operative fixation are any sagittal malalignment greater than 10° or 3–4 mm of displacement in any plane [2, 3]. Multiple metatarsal fractures may also be indicated for operative fixation; however, they will often move as a unit due to intermetatarsal ligaments [1].

Operative Events

About 6 weeks after the injury was sustained, the patient went to the operating room. Again, this delay was not ideal, but due to her difficulty getting to appointments to check her blisters, her surgery could not be set up in a timely manner. She underwent general anesthesia and a tourniquet was used on her right lower extremity. The skin incision was made on the dorsal aspect of the foot, between the second and third metatarsals. Dissection was carried down to the periosteum where abundant callus was found around the fracture sites. This was removed from the distal fractures of both metatarsals and the fracture ends were cleaned. The second metatarsal was fixed with a 2.5 mm 5-hole plate, which allowed screws to be inserted on both the proximal and distal portions of the bone without approaching the fracture line or joint surface. The third metatarsal fracture was pinned, using 0.062 in. double ended Kirschner wire, for reasons listed above. It was pinned using an antegrade-retrograde intramedullary technique. The pin started in the dorsal incision since it was already open, then exited the distal portion of the metatarsal followed by

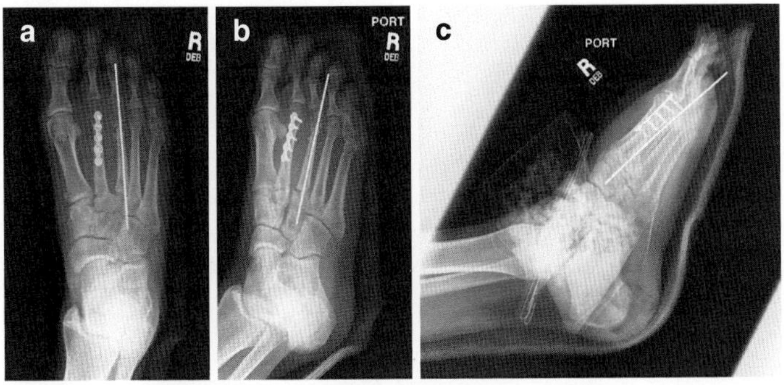

FIGURE 17.3 Right foot immediate postoperative radiographs. (**a**) (AP), (**b**) (oblique), (**c**) (lateral). The second metatarsal has interval placement of a 2.5 mm five-hole plate over the distal fracture. The third metatarsal has interval placement of an intramedullary pin, which extends to the body of the lateral cuneiform, due to the segmental nature of the fracture, and exits in the plantar foot. The foot is now in a posterior fiberglass splint

retrograde advancement of the distal portion of the pin into the proximal metatarsal. The proximal portion of the Kirschner wire extended to the body of the lateral cuneiform, because of the segmental nature of the fracture. The incisions were irrigated and closed (Fig. 17.3a–c).

Postoperative Plan

The patient's incisions were dressed and she was placed in a fiberglass posterior splint for protection with instructions for non-weight bearing on the right lower extremity. She was also given a prescription for aspirin 325 mg by mouth daily for 30 days for venous thromboembolism prophylaxis, as is the standard protocol at this particular institution. At 2 weeks postoperatively, her wounds were assessed as healing appropriately and her sutures were removed. She was to remain non-weight bearing in a splint. She had difficulty obtaining radiographs at this stage. At 5 weeks postoperatively, she still had difficulty obtaining radiographs, but her pin was removed

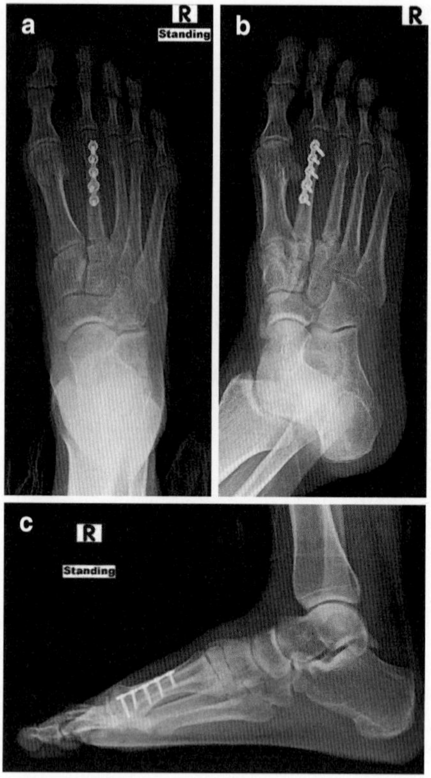

FIGURE 17.4 Right foot radiographs from 8 weeks postoperatively. (**a**) (AP), (**b**) (oblique), (**c**) (lateral). Second metatarsal plate in place. Interval removal of third metatarsal intramedullary pin. Alignment of metatarsals well maintained. Interval callus formation, but some fracture line still visible, particularly in the proximal fractures

at that point in time. She would continue non-weight bearing until radiographs could be obtained. She returned at 8 weeks postoperatively with radiographs (Fig. 17.4a–c) showing maintained alignment of the metatarsals with signs of appropriate healing. At this point her pain was much improved as well. She was made weight bearing as tolerated in a short walking boot and instructed to return in 6 weeks for final radiograph to ensure complete union of the fractures.

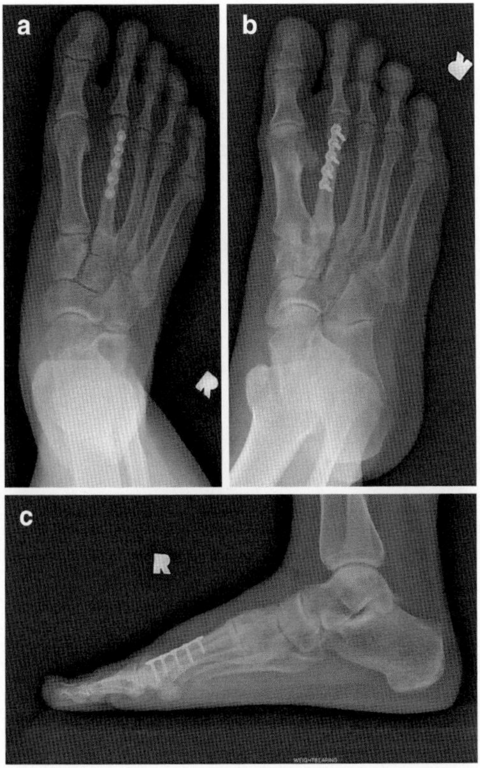

FIGURE 17.5 Right foot radiographs from 1 year postoperatively. (**a**) (AP), (**b**) (oblique), (**c**) (lateral). Second metatarsal plate in place with no implant migration. Fractures well healed with excellent alignment

Outcome

The patient had bilateral foot radiographs at her primary care physician's office due to nondescript bilateral foot pain during pregnancy about a year out from surgery. These show excellent alignment of the metatarsals with the plate in place and healed fracture lines (Fig. 17.5a–c).

Salient Points/Pearls

- Metatarsals have a significant degree of soft tissue attachments including muscles and ligaments; therefore the degree of displacement often correlates with the severity and energy level of the injury [4].
- Nondisplaced or minimally displaced metatarsal fractures are generally treated nonoperatively with immobilization and unloading of the metatarsals for 4–6 weeks. Unloading options will be determined by the patient's level of comfort and can range from compressive wraps to a short leg cast, but more commonly a hard soled shoe or a walking boot is utilized [4].
- Sagittal plane displacement may lead to malunion and metatarsalgia, particularly from prominent metatarsal heads. Transverse plane displacement and malunion may lead to symptomatic interdigital nerve compression or may disrupt the integrity of the forefoot arch, limiting activity [1–5]. This is reflected in general operative indications of sagittal malalignment greater than 10° or 3–4 mm of displacement in any plane [2, 3].
- Closed reduction and pinning are typically done with retrograde technique. In order to avoid rebound toe dorsiflexion, it is recommended to insert the pin through a plantarflexed proximal phalanx rather than the distal metatarsal. This method may lead to metatarsophalangeal stiffness, but it will prevent a dorsiflexion contracture at that joint [3].
- Antegrade pinning is an alternative option. This can be accomplished with a prebent wire to aid in reduction. The advantages are less stiffness at the metatarsophalangeal joint and earlier weight bearing (because the pins exit the skin dorsally rather than plantar). The prebent pin can pierce osteoporotic bone or patients with narrow medullary canals [5].
- Open reduction internal fixation with a plate, when compared to pinning, is associated with greater stability, less joint stiffness, and no pin site complications [4]. There are

low rates of incisional complications. In open cases, stripping of tissue can lead to devascularization. At times, as in the above case, one may be limited by the amount of available bone stock, and open reduction internal fixation may not even be an option [5].

- Despite the method of fixation, most metatarsal fractures lead to acceptable outcomes [5].

References

1. Sanders R, Papp S. Fractures of the midfoot and forefoot. In: Mann RA, Coughlin MJ, editors. Surgery of the foot and ankle. 8th ed. St Louis: Mosby; 2006. p. 2215–9.
2. Fetzer GB, Wright RW. Metatarsal shaft fractures and fractures of the proximal fifth metatarsal. Clin Sports Med. 2006;25(1):139–50.
3. Rammelt S, Heineck J, Zwipp H. Metatarsal fractures. Injury. 2004;35(Suppl 2):SB77–86.
4. Richter M, Kwon JY, DiGiovanni CW. Foot injuries. In: Browner BD, Jupiter JB, Krettek C, Anderson PA, editors. Skeletal trauma: basic science, management and reconstruction. 5th ed. Philadelphia: Elsevier; 2015. p. 2347–63.
5. Kim HN, Park YJ, Kim GL, Park YW. Closed antegrade intramedullary pinning for reduction and fixation of metatarsal fractures. J Foot Ankle Surg. 2012;51(4):445–9.

Chapter 18
Calcaneus Malunion with Subtalar Fusion (Bone Block Arthrodesis)

Selene G. Parekh and Rajiv Shah

Case Presentation

A 35-year-old male anesthetist fell from height 7 years ago. He sustained an intra-articular fracture of the right calcaneus. He was treated conservatively with a short leg cast for 6 weeks followed by mobilization. The patient had progressively worsening pain, swelling, and disfigurement in the ankle with a limp. He specifically complained of difficulty

S.G. Parekh, M.D., M.B.A. (✉)
Department of Orthopaedic Surgery, Duke University Medical Center, Durham, NC, USA
e-mail: selene.parekh@gmail.com

R. Shah, M.S. (Ortho)
Department of Foot and Ankle Orthopaedics, Sunshine Global Hospitals, Vadodara, India

N.C. Tejwani (ed.), *Fractures of the Foot and Ankle*,
DOI 10.1007/978-3-319-60456-5_18,

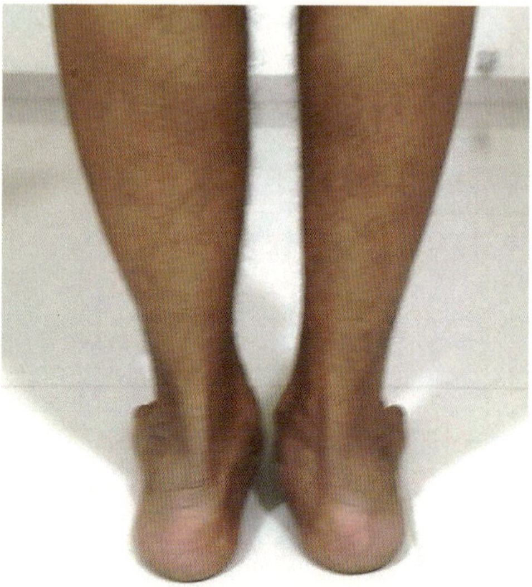

FIGURE 18.1 Standing clinical picture of a patient showing broadened right heel positioned in more valgus than left heel

with pain on walking on uneven grounds. His standing clinical picture from behind showed broadening, shortening, and valgus positioning of the right heel (Fig. 18.1).

Radiological Evaluation

Weight-bearing ankle and foot series X-rays were taken. The lateral film demonstrated shortening of the calcaneus, subtalar arthritis, and posterior exostosis from malunited calcaneus. The talus was dorsiflexed in the ankle mortise (Fig. 18.2). Comparative axial views were taken to judge the amount of heel shortening, broadening, and positioning of the heel. The heel was positioned in more valgus than the opposite side (Fig. 18.3).

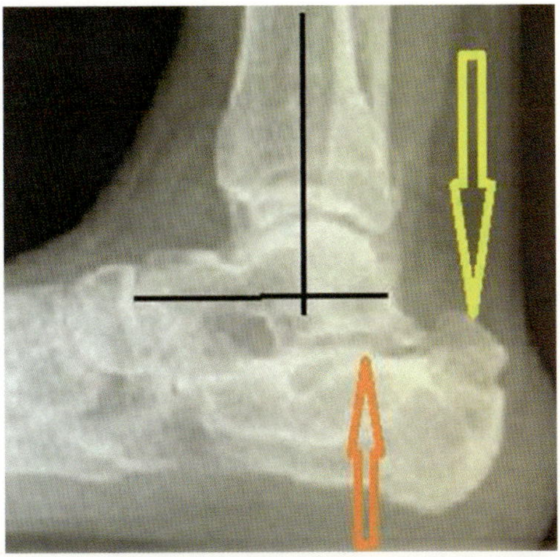

Figure 18.2 The lateral radiograph of the right heel showing subtalar arthritis (*orange arrow*) and posterior exostosis (*yellow arrow*). Note that talus is also dorsiflexed in the ankle mortise (*black lines*)

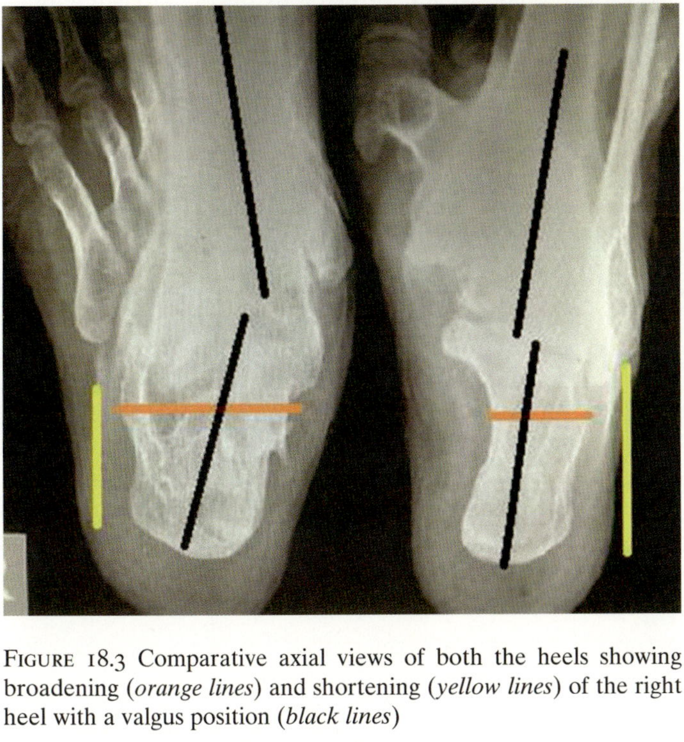

Figure 18.3 Comparative axial views of both the heels showing broadening (*orange lines*) and shortening (*yellow lines*) of the right heel with a valgus position (*black lines*)

Treatment

Surgery was planned after preoperative medical clearance. At surgery it was planned to perform a subtalar fusion with distraction bone grafting to treat the subtalar arthritis as well as the widening and shortening of the heel. The ipsilateral iliac crest was selected for tricortical bone graft harvesting. Bone graft placement was planned in such a manner to increase the height of posterior subtalar joint to address the talar dorsiflexion. The correction of the valgus heel was accomplished by carrying out generous soft-tissue releases and strategical shaping and placing of the bone graft. The lateral and posterior exostectomy was also planned together with these surgical procedures. The logic was to target all the pain-generating elements of the calcaneus malunion. The valgus positioning of heel was thought to get corrected by the generous release. If not able, a calcaneal osteotomy would be required.

Surgical Tact

Position

The patient was placed in a lateral decubitus position with affected lower limb facing up. Alternatively, a directly posterior approach can be used, with the patient in a prone position. The right limb was slightly flexed at the knee to bring the heel to the corner of the radiolucent table. A thigh tourniquet was applied and the ipsilateral iliac crest was also prepared (Fig. 18.4). An image intensifier was positioned diagonally in such a manner that an AP projection would show the lateral image of the calcaneus and a lateral projection would show an axial image of the calcaneus assisted by dorsiflexion of the foot (Fig. 18.5).

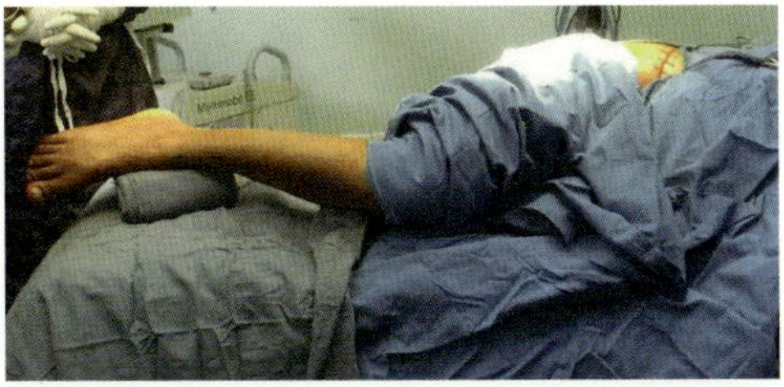

FIGURE 18.4 The patient position at surgery. The patient lies in a lateral decubitus position with affected limb up towards the ceiling. The ipsilateral iliac crest is also prepared

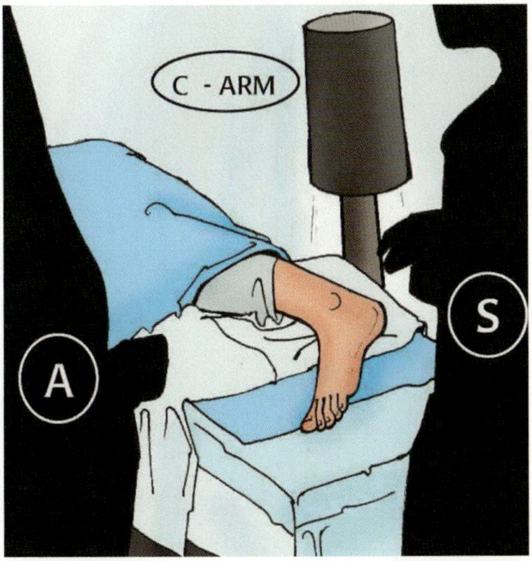

FIGURE 18.5 Positions of operative personnel at surgery. Surgeon stands at heel end of affected foot while assistant stands at the toe end with diagonally positioned image intensifier

Approach

A lateral extensile approach based on the lateral plantar artery was used (Fig. 18.6). The peroneals, calcaneo-fibular ligament, and sural nerve were lifted within the flap. The flap was handled gently with blunt skin hooks and the flap lifting was assisted with sharp dissection. The flap was retracted with two bent k-wires, one wire each in the anterior and posterior talus (Fig. 18.7). The flap was kept moist with the use of a wet gauze. This approach gave an access to the subtalar joint as well as the posterior exostosis. This approach would also allow for a medial calcaneal slide osteotomy, if at all it was needed.

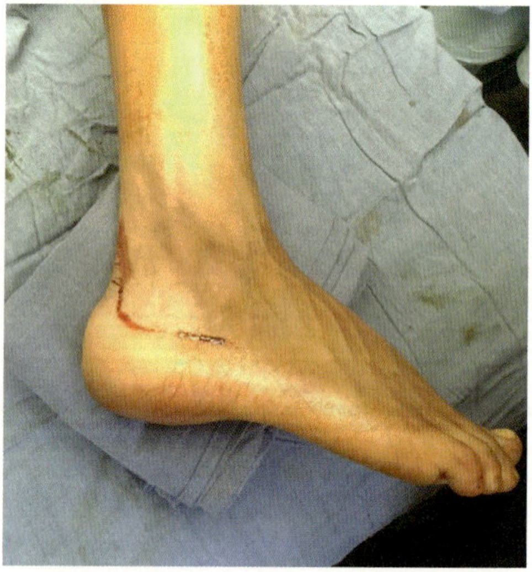

FIGURE 18.6 The lateral extensile approach

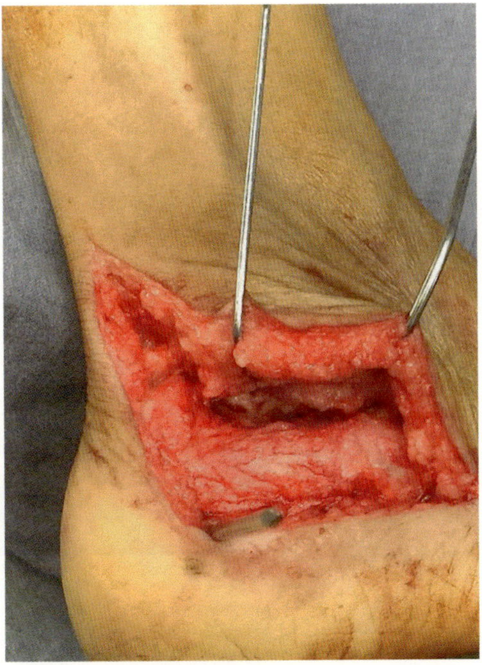

Figure 18.7 Positioning of two k-wires for retraction of the flap

Exostectomy

Exposure with extension of the proximal limb and retraction of the Achilles allowed for complete visualization of the lateral as well as posterior exostosis (Fig. 18.8). The lateral wall exostosis was resected flush with the lateral talar wall. With the heel in plantarflexion, the tendoachilles was retracted posteriorly and all prominent bone in front of it was excised taking care of not entering into the posterior subtalar joint (Fig. 18.9). Fluoroscopic imaging was used to verify the adequacy of this bone removal. The excised bone was preserved for utilization as bone graft in the subtalar distraction arthrodesis.

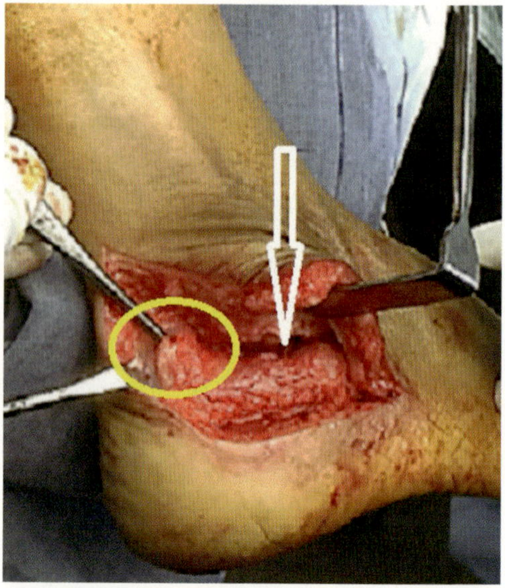

Figure 18.8 Demonstration of the lateral wall exostosis (*white arrow*) and posterior wall exostosis (*yellow circle*)

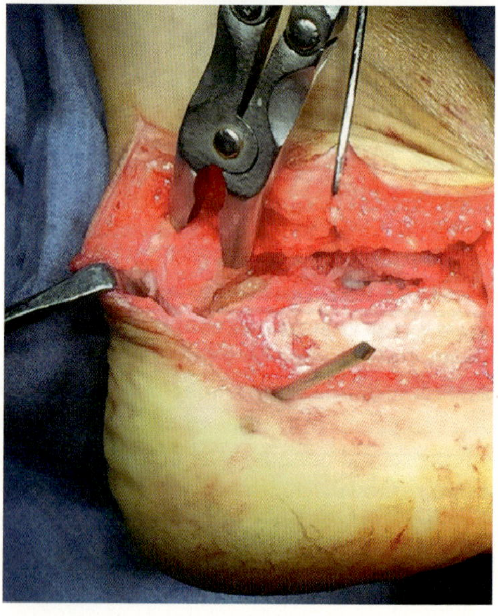

Figure 18.9 Excision and removal of posterior exostosis

Fusion and Fixation

Meticulous preparation of the subtalar joint articulating surfaces must be performed. The articular cartilage is denuded up to bleeding subchondral bone with curettes, osteotomes, or a saw. Infrequently, a burr is used, but care is taken to irrigate the burr to avoid any thermal necrosis of the bone. Visualization of the flexor hallucis longus marks the completion of joint preparation medially. This was followed by drilling of the subchondral bone and feathering of the articular margins to increase the bleeding bone surface area. Once the joint is prepared and mobilized, a laminar spreader in the joint, or a pin distraction, can help in distracting the joint and restoring the talar declination angle. An image is checked with the distracted lamina spreader to get a precise idea about restoration of heel height. After release of soft tissues, the subtalar joint and the heel could easily be manipulated out of gross valgus to neutral obviating the need for a medial slide calcaneal osteotomy. The graft size was measured. An adequately sized iliac crest bone graft was harvested and crafted to fit in the space created. The bone graft was positioned in the subtalar joint in such a manner that the posterior heel height could be restored, the hindfoot could be put out of valgus, and the talar declination angle could be improved. Additional cancellous graft from the iliac crest and from the excised bone was packed into the fusion site. At this stage, soft tissue-retracting k-wires were removed and flap closure assessment was done.

Guide wires for large cannulated screws were passed from the non-weight-bearing area of the heel up towards the talar neck in parallel fashion. These wires were placed medially and laterally under axial view guidance. Fluoroscopy was used to confirm their correct positioning followed by placement of 6.5–7.0 mm cannulated cancellous screws. After final image check with AP, lateral, axial, and Broden images, closure was performed. The flap was closed in two layers over a drain and compression dressings with plaster splintage were applied (Fig. 18.10).

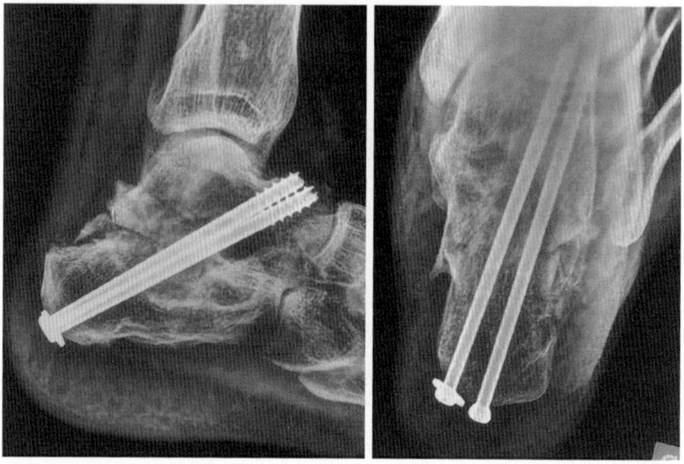

FIGURE 18.10 Lateral and axial postoperative image at the end of 5 months

Postoperative Plan

Sutures were removed between the 10th and 14th days and a below-the-knee cast was continued for a total of 4–6 weeks. The first radiological assessment was done at first visit, and another at the 6 weeks. The patient was allowed full weight bearing at the end of 8–10 weeks, in a boot, once enough bone was visualized on radiographs. Solid fusion is typically achieved 3–6 months after the surgery.

Outcome

The patient was relieved of anterior as well as subfibular pain. His plantarflexion was nearly normal with approximately 5° of dorsiflexion. There was a noticeable reduction in his limp and he could do all activities of his daily routine at the end of 3 months.

Subtalar distraction arthrodesis is known to provide high fusion rates and pain relief (Jackson JB 3rd, Jacobson L, Banerjee R, Nickisch F. Foot Ankle Clin. 2015 Jun;20(2):335–51. doi: 10.1016/j.fcl.2015.02.004. Epub 2015 Apr 11. Distraction subtalar arthrodesis.; Subtalar Distraction Arthrodesis with Fresh Frozen Femoral Neck Allograft: A Retrospective Case Series. Monaco SJ, Brandao RA, Manway JM, Burns PR. Foot Ankle Spec. 2016 Jul 1). A variety of distraction materials can be used, ranging from autograft, allograft, and even tantalum wedges successfully (Isolated Subtalar Distraction Arthrodesis Using Porous Tantalum: A Pilot Study. Papadelis EA, Karampinas PK, Kavroudakis E, Vlamis J, Polizois VD, Pneumaticos SG. Foot Ankle Int. 2015 Sep;36(9):1084–8). Minor wound complications are common; however significant improvement in patient outcomes scores can be expected (Foot (Edinb). 2013 Mar;23(1):39–44. doi: 10.1016/j.foot.2012.10.004. Epub 2012 Nov 21.

The subtalar distraction bone block arthrodesis following the late complications of calcaneal fractures: a systematic review. Schepers T.)

Salient Points/Pearls

- Calcaneal malunion cases present with a constellation of multiple problems with pain being the most common complaint [1–3]. Direct involvement of the subtalar and calcaneocuboid joints will lead to painful arthritis of both of these joints [1, 2]. Ankle joint may be secondarily involved due to a dorsiflexed talus in the ankle mortise leading to painful anterior ankle impingement and ankle arthrosis at a later date [1]. The calcaneus, being a subcutaneous bone, is surrounded by many important structures. Laterally, these include the peronei. Medially, there is the tendon of the flexor halluces and digitorum longus and branches of the posterior tibial nerve. Posteriorly there is the attachment of the Achilles tendon, while inferiorly, there is the heel fat pad. Malunions of the calcaneus with displaced bony fragments will generate secondary pressure effects on these surrounding structures like tendons, ligaments, and nerves leading to tenosynovitis, tendonitis, or tears of tendons and compressive neuropathy of adjacent nerves [1]. The sural and posterior tibial nerve may suffer traction or compression injuries in cases of calcaneal malunions [3]. In any given case of a calcaneal malunion, combinations of these malunion elements may be present. With the help of clinical as well as radiological examinations, the clinician should aim to find out every such pain-generating element (pain generators). Diagnostic injections in and around joints, nerves, and tendons could help in differentiating pain generators. These injections may be ultrasound guided or image guided.

- In the present case, pain generators included subtalar arthritis, posterior and lateral exostosis, talar dorsiflexion, heel shortening, and heel valgus. Hence surgery was planned to address each of these.
- As a routine practice, at the end of clinical and radiological evaluations, authors formulate a ten-point checklist which essentially guides towards precise planning of treatment. These ten checklist points are as follows:
  - Duration of malunion
  - Prior treatment
  - Position of previous scars
  - Presence of implants
  - Pressure areas and problems: Medial/lateral/posterior/plantar
  - Joint status: Calcaneocuboid/subtalar/talonavicular/ankle
  - Deformities: Forefoot/midfoot/hind foot
  - Status of tendons: TP/FHL/tendoachilles
  - Nerve pressure: Sural/posterior tibial/others
  - Quality of bone
- The treatment plan for calcaneus malunion is comprised of four major decisions:
  - Approach and incisions
  - Soft tissue procedures

- Bony procedures
- Order and staging of procedures

- Approach and incision: For dealing with cases with a large lateral wall exostosis and big shortening correction, the lateral extensile approach is preferred. Moreover, the ability to perform a calcaneal osteotomy can be conducted with this approach. In cases where closure difficulties are anticipated, a posterior or posterolateral approach may be preferred over the extensile lateral approach [4]. A minimally invasive sinus tarsi approach may be tried in selected cases with minimal shortening and the absence of deformity. In cases where a medial wall exostosis is present, signs and symptoms of secondary tarsal tunnel compression may be experienced. A separate medial approach may be required (Fig. 18.11) to decompress the nerve. The extensile lateral approach more often than not is adequate

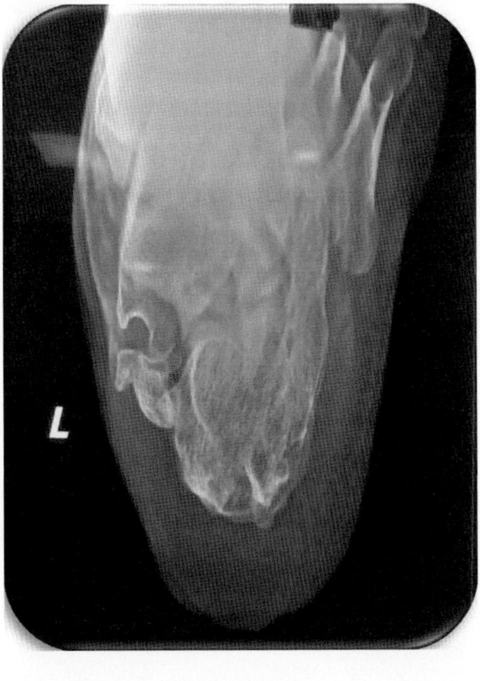

FIGURE 18.11 Calcaneus malunion case with medial exostosis and impingement which required separate medial approach

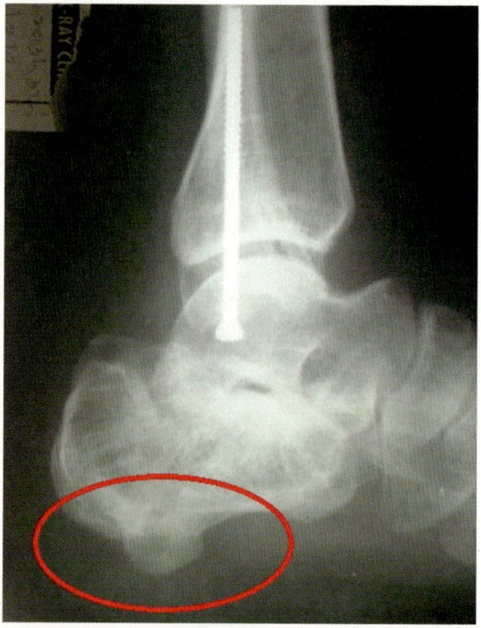

FIGURE 18.12 Case of plantar exostosis which required direct plantar approach for excision

for excision of the plantar exostosis. Very rarely is a separate plantar approach needed for excision of such plantar exostosis (Fig. 18.12).

- Soft tissue procedures: Very few malunion cases can easily be managed by lateral wall decompression alone. Soft tissue procedures, in the form of a tendon release, tenosynovectomy, nerve release, neurectomy, or nerve burial may be required as well [5]. Cases with the late effects of compartment syndrome in the form of claw toes would also need reconstructive procedures. In many cases, a triple hemi section lengthening of tendoachilles may be needed.
- Bony procedures: Bony procedures could be either joint sparing or joint sacrificing. An osteotomy below the subtalar joint, with correction of the heel height, can be used in mild cases with little or no arthritis and will spare the subtalar joint [6]. Excision of isolated exostosis is another joint-sparing procedure for extra-articualr malunion cases

[7]. Fusion of affected joints is the ultimate joint-sacrificing procedure. Fusions may be done in situ, in distraction with a bone block, and with the aid of corrective osteotomies [6, 7]. Romash described a corrective osteotomy through the original fracture with a subtalar fusion resulting in successful results [8]. A vertical slide osteotomy was described for cases where impingement of malleoli was found due to heel shortening. This osteotomy would not correct talar inclination and will not relieve anterior ankle impingement symptoms [9]. A fusion of the subtalar joint and tendoachilles lengthening is done in conjunction with this osteotomy [10] leading to an estimated 91% excellent results by Huang et al. [10]. Bone graft harvesting and arthrodesis and arthroplasty for claw toes are other examples of bony procedures.

- Order and staging of procedures: An osteotomy for correction of heel varus or valgus must follow joint preparation. Fixation of the osteotomy must precede the fusion procedure or be incorporated in the construct [9]. A plantar exostectomy must precede fixation. Medial exostectomy and decompression can be performed after the fusion procedures, as it requires turning the patient in a supine position. Reconstructive soft tissue and bony procedures for the midfoot and forefoot may be staged for another surgical sitting.
- Lui described the arthroscopic management of the late sequelae of calcaneal malunions. Procedures include the release of the calcaneo-fibular impingement, release of the calcaneocuboid impingement, and release of the posterior tendoachilles impingement with two- or three-portal endoscopy [11, 12]. Joint procedures include arthroscopic subtalar and calcaneocuboid fusions as well as arthrolysis of the subtalar joint for stiffness without arthritis. These are symptom-specific procedures and accurate diagnosis would only yield good end results. These technically demanding procedures do have a learning curve and limitations in cases with gross deformities [11].

References

1. Nickisch F, Anderson RB. Post-calcaneus fracture reconstruction. Foot Ankle Clin. 2006;11:85–103.
2. Pier CP, Enrico P, Paola A. Treatment of late complications of intra-articular calcaneal fractures. Clin Podiatr Med Surg. 2006;23:355–74.
3. Verrabdhadra R, Tomiko F, Amy JP. Calcaneus malunion and non-union. Foot Ankle Clin. 2007;12:125–35.
4. Myerson M, Quill G Jr. Late complications of fractures of the calcaneus. J Bone Joint Surg. 1993;75A(3):331–41.
5. Garras DN, Santangelo JR, Wang DW, Easley ME. Subtalar distraction using interpositional frozen structural allograft. Foot Ankle Int. 2008;29:561–72.
6. Stephens H, Sanders R. Calcaneal malunions: results of prognostic computed tomography classification system. Foot Ankle Int. 1996;17(7):395–401.
7. Braley WG, Bishop JO, Tullos HS. Lateral decompression for malunited os calcis fractures. Foot Ankle. 1985;6(2):90–6.
8. Clare MP, Lee WE 3rd, Sanders RW. Intermediate to long term results of a treatment protocol for calcaneus fracture malunions. J Bone Joint Surg Am. 2005;87(5):963–73.
9. Guang-Rong Y, Sun-Jun HU, Yang Y-F, Zhao H-M, Zhang S-M. Reconstruction of calcaneus fracture malunion with osteotomy and subtalar joint salvage: technique and outcomes. Foot Ankle Int. 2013;34:726–32.
10. Romash MM. Reconstructive osteotomy of the calcaneus with subtalar arthrodesis for malunited calcaneal fractures. Clin Orthop Relat Res. 1993;(290):157–67.
11. Huang PJ, YC F, Cheng YM, Lin SY. Subtalar arthrodesis for late sequelae of calcaneal fractures: fusion in situ versus fusion with sliding corrective osteotomy. Foot Ankle Int. 1999;20(3):166–70.
12. Lui TH. Posterior ankle impingement syndrome caused by malunion of joint depressed type calcaneal fracture. Knee Surg Sports Traumatol Arthrosc. 2008;16:687–9.

Chapter 19
Nail Plate Combination (NPC) Treatment for Infected, Charcot Ankle Fracture Malunion

Nicole M. Stevens, Richard S. Yoon, and Frank A. Liporace

Case Presentation

This is a 56-year-old female with past medical history significant for diabetes mellitus that sustained a trip and fall from standing height. Prior to her injury, she walked at baseline with a rolling walker. She is an insulin-dependent diabetic with poor control (last Hemoglobin A1c: 9.3) and bilateral peripheral neuropathy at baseline.

Initial Injury films (Fig. 19.1a–c) exhibit a left trimalleolar ankle fracture.

Initial Management and Treatment Course Until Malunion: Definitive fixation was performed on post-injury day 4, when

N.M. Stevens, M.D.
Department of Orthopaedic Surgery, NYU Hospital for Joint Diseases, 301 E 17th Street, Suite 1402, New York, NY, USA

R.S. Yoon, M.D. • F.A. Liporace, M.D. (✉)
Department of Orthopaedic Surgery, Jersey City Medical Center—RWJBarnabas Health, 355 Grand Street, Jersey City, NJ, USA
e-mail: liporace33@gmail.com

N.C. Tejwani (ed.), *Fractures of the Foot and Ankle*,
DOI 10.1007/978-3-319-60456-5_19,

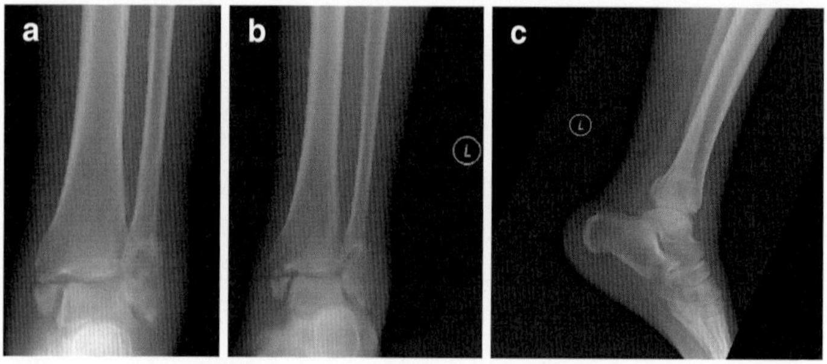

FIGURE 19.1 (**a**) AP, (**b**) mortise, and (**c**) lateral radiographs of initial unstable trimalleolar ankle fracture

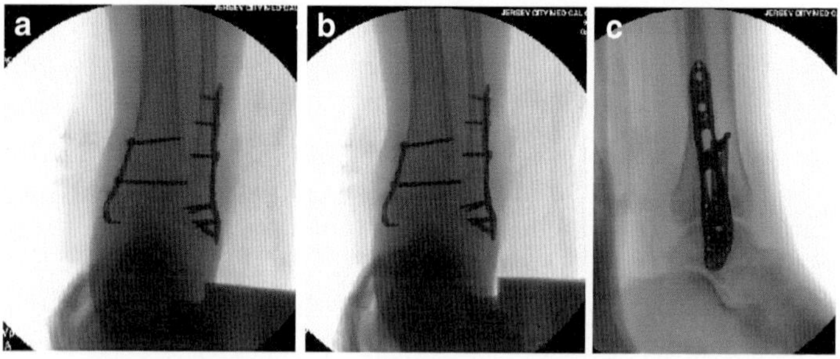

FIGURE 19.2 (**a**) AP, (**b**) mortise, and (**c**) lateral intraoperative fluoroscopy of primary fixation showing a bridge plate spanning the comminuted fibula fracture and an anti-glide plate reducing the medial malleolus

the soft tissues were deemed amenable to surgery. Patient underwent uneventful open reduction and fixation (ORIF) of both the fibular and medial malleolus. Intraoperatively, a vertical extension of the medial malleolar fracture was identified, and thus, an anti-glide construct was used with a plate; intraoperative external rotation stress was negative (Fig. 19.2a–c). The patient tolerated her surgery well and was discharged to a skilled nursing facility on postoperative day 3. The patient returned for her first postoperative visit at the 3-week time-point, when her wounds were healed and sutures removed. At this time, she was casted with the plan of being non-weight bearing for a minimum of 12 weeks. However, after her first follow-up appointment, she was lost to follow-up until the 7-month time-point and had been non-compliant with weight bearing precautions.

Work-Up and Arriving at the Correct Diagnosis: Due to her neuropathy, the patient experienced minimal pain and thus was noncompliant with weight bearing precautions. She eventually eroded through her cast, which was self-discontinued at home. She returned to the office noting intermittent warmth and swelling of her left lower extremity.

Laboratory work-up revealed a slightly elevated white blood cell count (12.5 g/mcL, ref. range: 4.5–11.5 g/mcL) with elevated inflammatory markers (ESR 45, ref. range 0–10; CRP 110, ref. range 0–7). Joint aspiration confirmed suspicion of infection with a cell count of 75 K and 92% PMNs; cultures grew out methicillin-sensitive Staph Aureus (MSSA).

Radiographs revealed complete fixation failure of the medial side with concomitant joint space obliteration in the midst of an ongoing Charcot arthropathy (Fig. 19.3a–c). Closer examination of the radiographs reveals not only a complete loss of height (Fig. 19.3c), but also severe shortening of the entire hindfoot complex due to the bony destruction of the talus, as seen on the mortise view (Fig. B). The AP

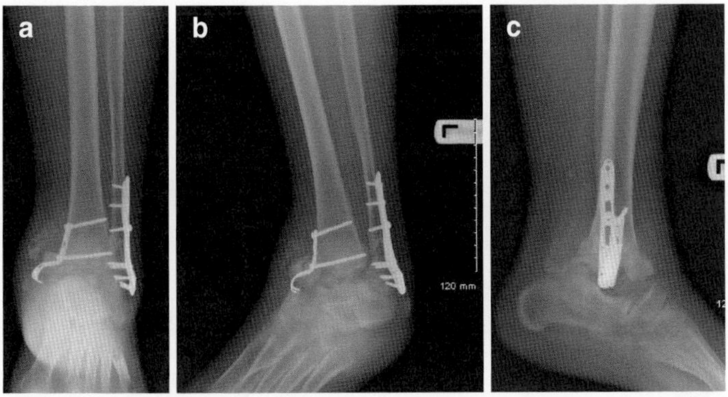

FIGURE 19.3 (**a**) AP, (**b**) mortise, and (**c**) lateral radiographs displaying failure of fixation, infected non-union, and Charcot arthropathy, of the ankle joint 7 months after primary fixation. The talus is obliterated, resulting in a loss of height and shortening of the hindfoot. Medialization of the hindfoot can also be appreciated on the AP view

view (Fig. 19.3a) shows medialization of the hindfoot complex in relation to the tibia further adding to the deformity. At this juncture, this patient had an infected ankle fracture malunion with significant deformity, namely loss of height, hindfoot shortening, and valgus deformity.

Staged Treatment Leading Up to Definitive Surgery: Initial treatment required urgent irrigation and debridement (I&D), removal of hardware, placement of an antibiotic spacer, and 6 weeks of intravenous (IV) antibiotics. During this initial ,debridement, care was taken to plan for the definitive surgery and utilizing incisions that would be used again. Furthermore, the goals of anatomic restoration of the deformity were applied during this stage (fibular and tibial osteotomy through the medial malleolus). Through a direct anterior approach, the remaining portion of the eroded medial malleolus was resected and all necrotic, infected tissue removed along with the hardware. A large enough antibiotic spacer (created with vancomycin/tobramycin in a 3:2 ratio) was made not only to restore height but overall length, which was maintained with an antibiotic tibiotalocalcaneal (TTC) nail prior to spacer placement (Fig. 19.4a–c). The patient

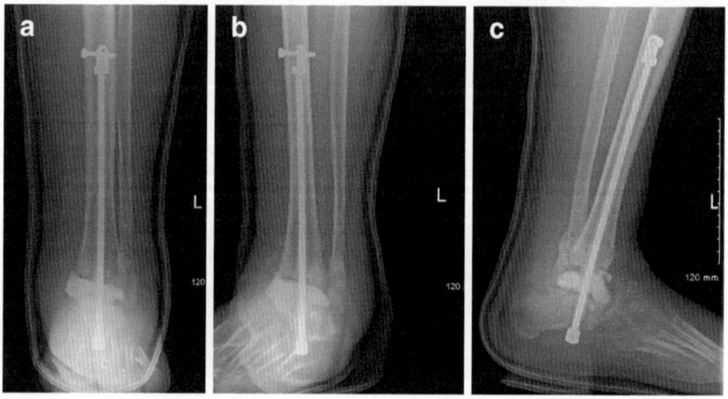

FIGURE 19.4 (**a**) AP, (**b**) mortise, and (**c**) lateral postoperative radiographs displaying antibiotic coated intramedullary nail and antibiotic spacer with restoration of hindfoot length, limb height, and coronal deformity

tolerated the procedure well, made non-weight bearing, casted, and was treated with oxacillin 2 g IV q24 h for 6 weeks. Inflammatory markers down-trended during this time period and after a 2-week antibiotic holiday, repeat joint aspiration was negative. She was deemed to be ready for definitive treatment.

Surgical Tact

Position: Supine, bilateral Iliac crest.

Approach: Direct anterior, Retrograde TTC nail.

Ankle and Hindfoot Fusion with Extension to the Navicular and **Iliac Crest Autograft**: First, the direct anterior approach was performed in order to remove the antibiotic cement spacer. Care was taken to preserve the membrane that had formed around the cement spacer and using osteotomes, the cement spacer was carefully removed. The antibiotic rod was left in place in order to maintain tibial-calcaneal height. Next, the anterior-posterior shortening of the calcaneus/hindfoot complex was addressed. Two large laminar spreaders were utilized to bring out the length and confirmed on fluoroscopic imaging. Provisional fixation was done using 2.0 mm Kirschner wires placed percutaneously from distal to proximal in multiple planes. Next, two locking midfoot fusion plates were custom contoured to the patient's anatomy and placed from the tibia to the talus anterolaterally, and from the tibia to the navicular anteromedially. Care was taken to place screws around the antibiotic rod in order to create a corridor for the eventual TTC nail [1–4]. With the hindfoot length addressed, attention was turned to the tibial-calcaneal height and valgus deformity. The custom contoured plates also functioned to temporarily hold the extremity height—allowing removal of the antibiotic rod. Once the antibiotic rod was removed, the remaining cartilage and nonviable bone was excised. The bony defect was measured and bilateral iliac crest cortical bone grafts were harvested to adequately fill the space and provide compressive strength. The iliac crest bone graft was wedge fit underneath the two

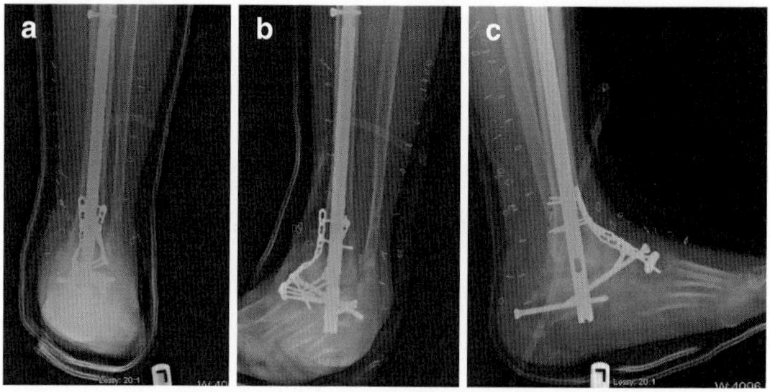

FIGURE 19.5 (**a**) AP, (**b**) mortise, and (**c**) lateral postoperative radiographs after definitive fixation displaying intramedullary retrograde tibiotalocalcaneal nail and two bridge plates to the navicular. The limb height, coronal alignment, and hindfoot length are maintained

precontoured plates to avoid graft dislodgement during placement of the TCC nail. After careful reaming, the TCC nail was inserted next, using a calcaneal start point, thus definitively addressing the height deformity. The nail was long enough to surpass all previous fixation and the isthmus of the bone, to avoid the creation of stress risers. Additionally, a 6.5 mm fully threaded screw was placed in a retrograde fashion from the navicular to the calcaneus around the nail to act as a post to help maintain the restored length. Once all hardware was in place, demineralized bone matrix, cancellous iliac crest autograft, and 1 gm of vancomycin powder were used to fill the remaining dead space. The membrane was approximated with 1-0 vicryl suture, and subsequent closure with 2-0 vicryl and 2-0 nylons for the skin was placed. The patient was placed in a circumferential negative pressure wound dressing and splinted in neutral dorsiflexion (Fig. 19.5a–c).

Postoperative Plan: The patient remained in a short leg splint and made non-weight bearing for a period of 12 weeks. Sutures were removed at 3 weeks. The patient's bony healing progressed well (6 weeks, Fig. 19.6a–c). As noted by the broken hardware by the time of consolidation

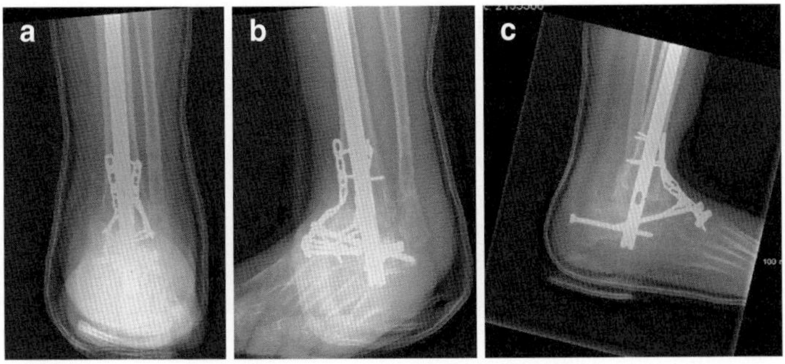

FIGURE 19.6 (**a**) AP, (**b**) mortise, and (**c**) lateral radiographs at 6 weeks postoperatively with well-aligned hardware and maintenance of reduction

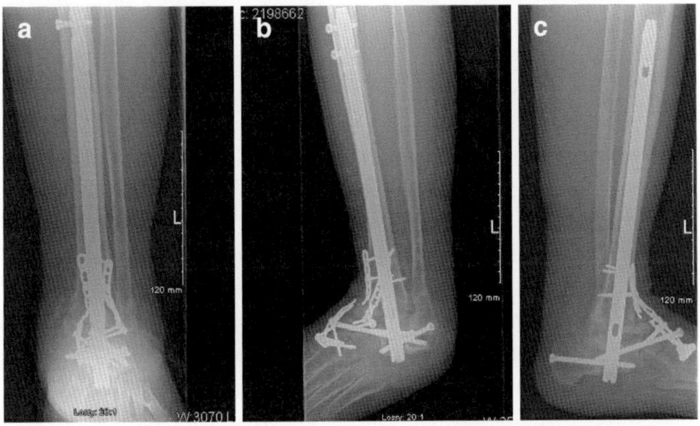

FIGURE 19.7 (**a**) AP, (**b**) mortise, and (**c**) lateral radiographs at 3 months displaying ankle fusion, with acceptable alignment. Note, the patient was likely walking on her affected extremity, indicated by a broken plate

(12 weeks, Fig. 19.7a–c), it had been clear that she had also been walking on the affected extremity. However with the stability of the construct, she maintained height and length and went onto uncomplicated fusion.

Complications: None. No plans for hardware removal.

Salient Points/Pearls

- Rates of complications and fracture fixation failure are high in diabetic patients—particularly among those with neuropathy [5]. They should be closely monitored postoperatively and may require longer periods of protected weight bearing, but still can fail.
- Always consider infection, and it must be ruled out prior to the next stage of surgery. This can be accomplished using serum WBC, ESR, CRP, aspiration cell count and culture (following a 2-week antibiotic holiday), and general clinical appearance.
- Plan incisions, deformity corrections, and constructs for future definitive procedures when performing temporizing procedures, like removal of hardware or spacer placement.
- Using temporizing fixation to correct deformity can make your second surgery easier.
- Additional plate fixation to maintain desired length and foot position in relation to the tibial axis not only protects against noncompliance but also acts as a "tension band" when placed anteriorly counteracting the pull of the Achilles' tendon, compressing the hindfoot fusion further [6].
- Be liberal with bone graft when fusing joints, remember to prep out both iliac crests for large defects.
- Fusion of Charcot joints should extend outside the area of Charcot arthropathy, which is why the navicular was included in this construct.

References

1. Paola LD, Volpe A, Varotto D, Postorino A, Brocco E, Enesi A, Merico M, de Vido D, da Ros R, Assaloni R. Use of a retrograde nail for ankle arthrodesis in Charcot Neuroarthropathy: a limb salvage procedure. Foot Ankle Int. 2007;28:967–70.
2. Qui GE. Reconstruction of Multiplanar ankle and Hindfoot deformity with intramedullary techniques. Foot Ankle Clin. 2009;14:533–47.

3. Rammelt S, Pyrc J, Agren PH, Hartstock LA, Cronier P, Friscia DA, Hansen ST, Schaser K, Ljungvist J, Sands AK. Tibiotalocalcaneal fusion using the Hindfoot arthrodesis nail: a multicenter study. Foot Ankle Int. 2013;34:1245–55.
4. Siebachmeyer M, Boddu K, Bilal A, Hester TW, Hardwick T, Fox TP, Edmonds M, Kavarthapu V. Outcomes of one stage correction of deformities of the ankle and hindfoot and fusion in Charcot neuroarthropathy using a retrograde intramedullary hindfoot arthrodesis nail. Bone Joint J. 2015;97:76–82.
5. Wukich DK, Joseph A, Ryan M, Ramirez C, Irrgang JJ. Outcomes of ankle fractures in patient with uncomplicated versus complicated diabetes. Foot Ankle Int. 2011;32:120–30.
6. Yoon RS, Bible J, Marcus MS, Donegan DJ, Bergmann KA, Siebler JC, Mir HR, Liporace FA. Outcomes following combined intramedullary nail and plate fixation for complex tibia fractures: a multicenter study. Injury. 2015;46:1097–101.

Chapter 20
Failed Syndesmotic Injury of Ankle

J. Dheenadhayalan

Case Presentation

The patient is a 27-year-old male who sustained an injury to his right ankle following a road traffic accident. He was evaluated in the emergency room and was noted to have a closed injury with no distal neurovascular deficit. His ankle was reduced and placed in a below knee splint.

Injury Films Taken before Splinting

Injury X-rays of the ankle (Fig. 20.1—anteroposterior and lateral views) show lateral malleolus fracture with subluxation of ankle joint, transverse medial malleolus fracture, and

J. Dheenadhayalan, M.S. (Ortho)
Department of Orthopaedics, Ganga Hospital, Coimbatore, India
e-mail: dheenu.dhayalan@gmail.com

N.C. Tejwani (ed.), *Fractures of the Foot and Ankle*,
DOI 10.1007/978-3-319-60456-5_20,

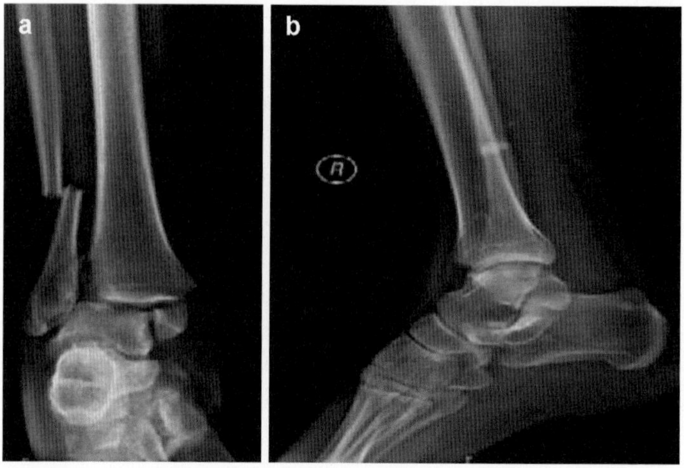

FIGURE 20.1 Shows anteroposterior and lateral views of ankle joint. (**a**). Anteroposterior view. (**b**). Lateral view

syndesmotic injury. Based on the Lauge Hansen classification this was a pronation external rotation injury (PER 4).

Using the Weber classification, this would be Type C indicating syndesmotic injury with the fracture of the fibula proximal to the syndesmosis.

Operative Treatment and Timing of Surgery

These injuries are generally associated with gross swelling and blisters may develop indicating more severe soft tissue damage. In case of gross swelling it is safe practice to wait till the appearance of wrinkle sign; meanwhile the joint can be stabilized with joint spanning external fixator if needed for stability.

However in this, the patient was seen immediately after injury and reduced, with minimal swelling observed.

As this was an unstable ankle fracture with joint subluxation, we decided to treat this fracture with open reduction and internal fixation with fibular plate, tension band wiring for medial malleolus, and screw fixation for syndesmotic injury [1].

Initial Surgery

- Lateral malleolus is fixed with 1/3rd tubular plate and medial malleolus with tension band wiring.
- For the syndesmotic injury, syndesmotic screw was placed from anterior to posterior direction.
- There is anterolateral bony fragment which was not fixed.
- Postoperative anteroposterior radiological report (Fig. 20.2) showed syndesmotic injury that was not reduced which can be determined by tibiofibular clear space >5 mm, tibiofibular overlap < 10 mm, and widened medial clear space. Therefore surgery was revised.

We believe that this was secondary to surgical error in not recognizing and reducing the syndesmosis. The bony fragment represents avulsion of the anterior tibiofibular ligament (ATFL) and should be recognized and reduced with fixation using a screw if the fragment is large enough.

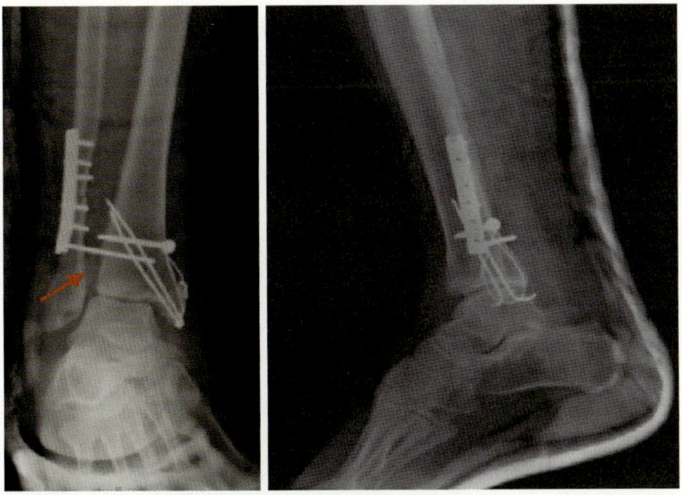

FIGURE 20.2 Shows avulsion of anterior tibiofibular ligament as evidenced by tibiofibular clear space >5 mm, tibiofibular overlap < 10 mm, and widened medial clear space

Also, in this case the syndesmosis screw is directed posteriorly likely exaggerating the mal-reduction by pushing the fibula posteriorly.

Postoperative Radiographs After First Surgery

After discussion with the patient, a repeat surgery was planned for reduction and fixation of the syndesmosis [2].

Surgical Technique

Position: Supine with sand bag under ipsilateral hip (Fig. 20.3).
Approach: Lateral approach over right ankle, using the distal end of the prior incision [4].

Fracture Reduction

The hardware for fixation of the malleoli was maintained as the fractures were deemed to be in acceptable position and

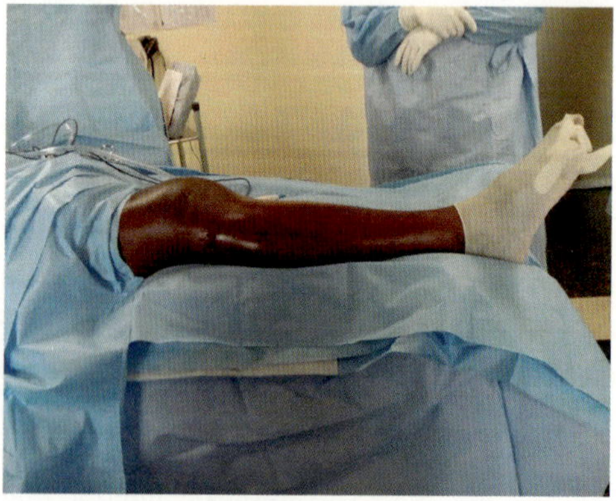

FIGURE 20.3 Shows supine position with pillow underneath the gluteal region to keep the limb in internal rotation for lateral approach of fibula

did not interfere with syndesmotic reduction. The mal-positioned syndesmotic screw was first removed.

An incision was made along the subcutaneous border of lateral malleolus. The syndesmosis was visualized and the bony fragment was reduced. The piece was too small to afford fixation; however once reduced, it was a guide to our reduction. A K-wire was used for holding the reduction of the piece (Fig. 20.4).

Use of a pointed reduction clamp was useful to allow reduction of the syndesmosis; care should be taken not to mal-reduce the syndesmosis. Placing the clamp tines in the same orientation as the syndesmosis is helpful along with direct visualization of the same [5].

Under c arm guidance syndesmotic injury was reduced with pointed reduction clamps with K-wire placed to hold the fixation temporarily. Fixation was achieved with two cortical screws with quadri-cortical purchase using 3.5 mm cortical screws [1].

Final radiographs show syndesmotic injury was reduced with implants in position. the reduction was confirmed by observing the tibiofibular overlap of >6mm and medial clear space of <4mm.(Figs. 20.4 and 20.5).

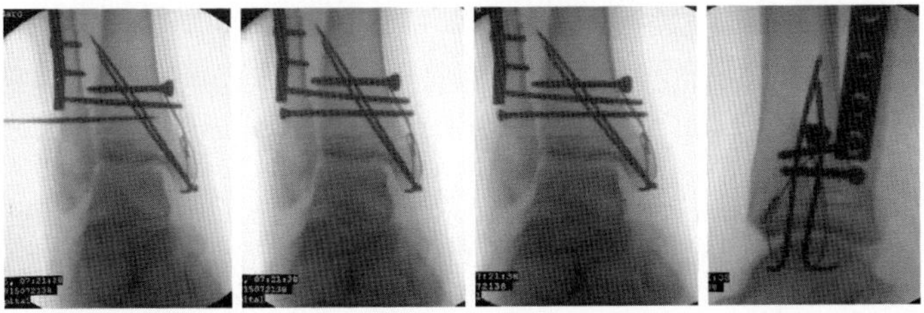

FIGURE 20.4 Shows that reduction is achieved after removal of the avulsed fragment, tibiofibular clear space, and overlap found to be in normal limits

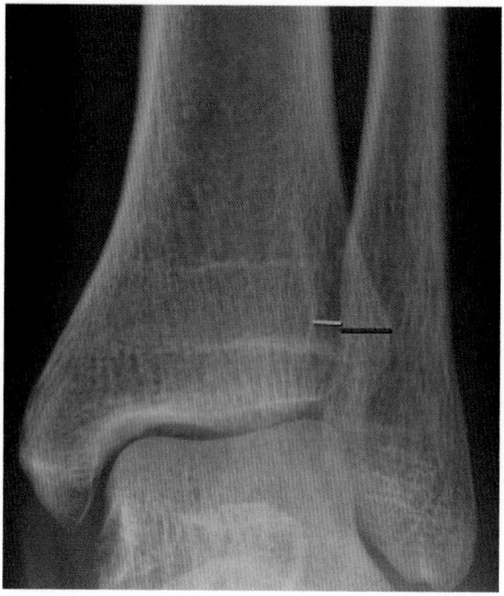

FIGURE 20.5 Shows a representative radiograph of tibiofibular overlap normal value >10mm (*red line*) and tibiofibular clear space normal value <5mm (*yellow line*)

Intraoperative Pictuires

Postoperative Plan

A below knee slab was placed for 6 weeks for the fracture to heal. The patient was allowed to do non-weight bearing during this time period.

After that the patient will be allowed to do partial and then full weight bearing as tolerated and physiotherapy for ankle range of motion as well.

Clinical and radiographic follow-up will be done till union, which was achieved without any further complications.

Expected Complications

Infection, implant failure, and ankle arthritis.

Salient Points/Pearls

- Syndesmotic injuries if diagnosed should be properly reduced and fixed with cortical screws along with fixation of bimalleolar fracture during surgery.
- Fixation of the fibula should be done first with one third tubular plate and the medial malleolus fixation with tension band wiring and K-wires or malleolar screws.
- Syndesmotic screw placement should be 2 cm above ankle joint and screws should be directed 30° anteriorly from fibula with ankle in neutral dorsiflexion [3] (Fig. 20.6). Talus, is shaped like a truncated cone and is wider anteriorly than posteriorly. Therefore in ankle dorsiflexion, fibula rotates externally through the tibiofibular syndesmosis, to accommodate this widened anterior surface of the talar dome.

Common errors in syndesmotic reduction are lack of recognition of the plane of the tibia-fibular joint; anterior or posterior mal-reduction due to improper clamp placement; incorrect screw orientation; and failure to appreciate the reduction (tibiofibular overlap and clear space)

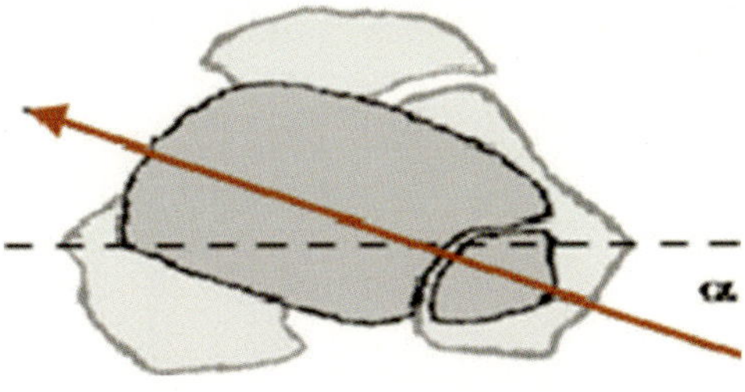

FIGURE 20.6 Posterior to anterior direction of syndesmotic screw. After reduction of the fibula at the syndesmosis, introduce the positioning screw obliquely from posterior to anterior at an angle of 25–30° and parallel to the tibial plafond

- Postoperatively non-weight bearing with walker for first 6 weeks and then gradually to partial and full weight bearing based on clinical and radiological findings.

References

1. Mosier-LaClair S, Pike H, Pomeroy G. Syndesmosis injuries: acute, chronic, new techniques for failed management. Foot Ankle Clin. 2002;7:551–65.
2. Parlamas G, Hannon C, Murawski G, et al. Treatment of chronic Syndesmotic injury: a systematic review and meta-analysis. Knee Surg Sports Traumatol Arthrosc. 2013;21(8):1931–9.
3. www2.aofoundation.org/wps/portal/surgerymobile?contentUrl=/srg/44/05-RedFix/Op/PosScrew/44-C2_PosScrw_2.jsp&soloState
4. Olson KM, Dairyko GH Jr, Toolan BC. Salvage of chronic instability of the syndesmosis with distal tibiofibular arthrodesis: functional and radiographic results. J Bone Joint Surg Am. 2011;93(1):66–72.
5. Zamzami MM. Chronic isolated distal tibiofibular syndesmotic disruption: diagnosis and management. Foot Ankle Surg. 2009;15:14–9.

Chapter 21
Charcot Arthropathy

Natalie R. Danna and Kenneth J. Mroczek

Case Presentation

The patient is a 52-year-old female with diabetes mellitus and neuropathy who presents with a progressive left ankle deformity over the last 2 years. She wears an Arizona brace for support.

Examination revealed a severe varus deformity at the ankle. She had palpable pulses and monofilament testing was consistent with neuropathy. Laterally, a 3 cm callus was present, but there was no ulceration or signs of infection. There was also no erythema or warmth.

N.R. Danna, M.D.
Department of Orthopedics, NYU Langone Medical Center, New York, NY, USA

K.J. Mroczek, M.D. (✉)
Department of Orthopedic Surgery, New York University Langone Hospital for Joint Diseases, 301 East 17th Street Suite 1616, New York, NY, USA
e-mail: kenneth.mroczek@nyumc.org

N.C. Tejwani (ed.), *Fractures of the Foot and Ankle*, DOI 10.1007/978-3-319-60456-5_21,

Initial Films

Standing films of the ankle (AP, lateral, mortise) and foot (AP, lateral, mortise) were obtained. They demonstrated a medial dislocation of the tibiotalar joint with diffuse osteopenia, nearly complete osteolysis of the talus, sclerosis, and osseous fragmentation (Figs. 21.1a–c and 21.2a–c).

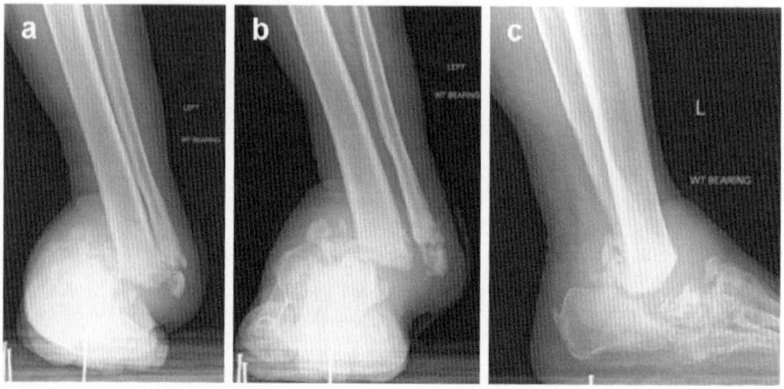

FIGURE 21.1 (**a–c**) Initial standing films of the ankle

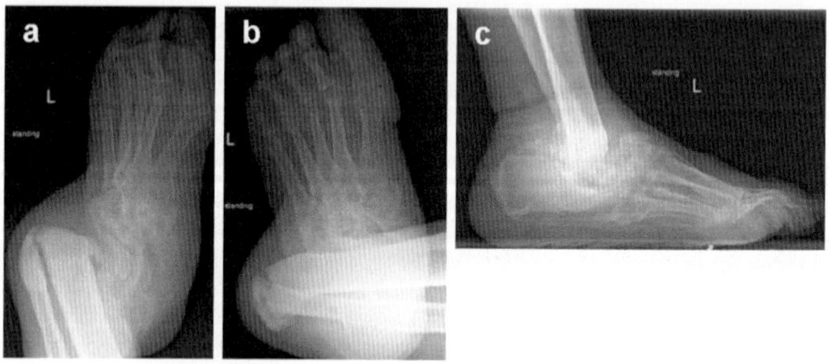

FIGURE 21.2 (**a–c**) Initial standing films of the foot

Treatment Considerations

Charcot neuroarthropathy occurs in patients with peripheral neuropathy, most commonly due to diabetes. It is a destructive process with potentially devastating results that can lead to significant deformity, ulceration, infection, and even amputation [1]. Charcot is often confused with an infection, but one must realize that an underlying infection is relatively uncommon in a patient without an ulcer or a history of an ulcer [2]. If concomitant osteomyelitis is suspected, a MRI with contrast is indicated. The MRI will most likely show marrow edema, especially in the acute phase, but the findings are only consistent with osteomyelitis if there is an ulcer in communication with the bone marrow edema.

Immobilization and offloading are the mainstays of treatment in the early stages [1]. This is usually achieved with a total contact cast or a pneumatic CAM boot [3]. Significant activity modification should be recommended, and a period of nonweightbearing can be considered depending on the acuity [4]. The goal of the immobilization is to provide support so that the patient will advance from the acute fragmentation phase to the consolidation phase.

If the patient progresses to the consolidation phase without significant deformity, then a custom brace or orthosis is recommended [3]. If they are consolidated and have a minor deformity with a prominence that leads to ulceration, then an irrigation, debridement, or partial ostectomy is recommended [4]. A course of culture-specific antibiotics should also be administered postoperatively. If the ulceration is located on the plantar surface, then the patient should be examined for an equinus contracture and an Achilles lengthening should be performed in addition to the ostectomy [1].

Patients who develop significant deformities require corrective fusions. If there is an infection or ulceration, then external fixation should be utilized. In all other cases, internal fixation is the best option since it is biomechanically stronger. A standard tibiotalar fusion is usually not possible due to extensive bony destruction with avascularity or necrosis common, particularly of the talus. As a result, the surgeon must be ready to extend the fusion to the calcaneus. Extending the fusion across the subtalar joint may also allow for stronger fixation and lessen the chance of failure. If the talus is completely necrotic, then a talectomy is indicated, and a tibiocalcaneal fusion would be performed [5]. Moreover, the degree of deformity may require extending to a tibiotalocalcaneal or even a pantalar fusion. The fixation can be performed using plates, cannulated screws, or an intramedullary nail. A combination of these fixation methods can also be utilized and is at the discretion of the surgeon. Regardless of the choice of fixation, more fixation than usual is recommended due to the poor quality of bone and possibility of hardware failure.

Patients must understand the severity of their condition and adhere to the prescribed postoperative protocol. In many cases, the patient may be nonweightbearing for 2–3 months. Strict glycemic control is advised. The cessation of smoking is mandatory. Realistic expectations and the possibility of a permanent brace must be discussed with the patient. Lastly, the possibility of failure and the need for amputation should also be addressed with the patient.

Surgical Tact

The patient underwent talectomy and tibiocalcaneal fusion with plate fixation. The fusion was supplemented with iliac crest aspirate, distal fibula autologous bone graft, and an implantable bone stimulator (Fig. 21.3a–c).

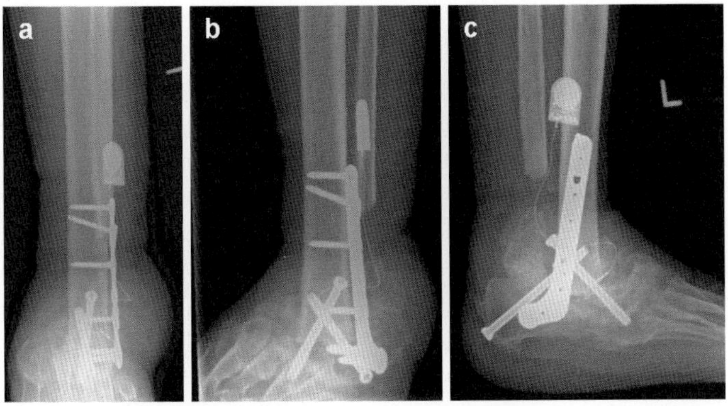

FIGURE 21.3 (**a**–**c**) Immediate postoperative films

Technique Specifics

The patient was placed in a semilateral decubitus position on a beanbag for the procedure, with the mini C-arm positioned on the ipsilateral side. The ankle was accessed laterally, through a lateral extensile approach. In this case, the majority of the talus was fragmented and eroded, so the devitalized bone was excised, leaving the tibia directly opposed to the calcaneus. The tibial and calcaneal surfaces were prepared with a sagittal saw. Two 8.0 mm crossed cannulated screws were used to achieve compression across the fusion mass. An (Integra Advansys) tibiocalcaneal plate was placed and fixed laterally. An excised segment of the fibula was morselized for bone graft and saturated with concentrated iliac crest bone marrow aspirate.

Postoperative Plan

The patient was made nonweightbearing in a short-leg cast for a period of 12 weeks. At this time, consolidation of the fusion mass was seen (Fig. 21.4a–c). Then the patient was made weightbearing as tolerated in a total contact cast for an additional 2 months before transitioning to a Charcot restraint

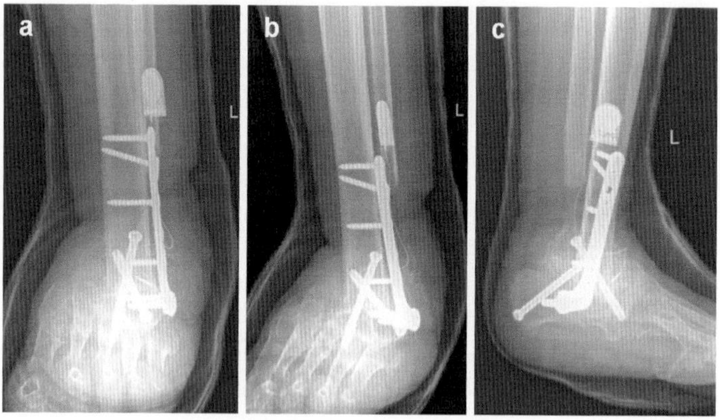

FIGURE 21.4 (**a–c**) 12-week postoperative films

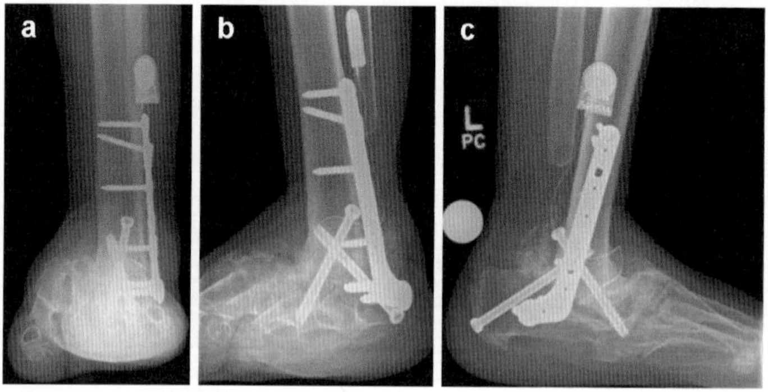

FIGURE 21.5 (**a–c**) 15-month postoperative films showing consolidation of the fusion and preserved alignment

orthotic walker (CROW) boot. At 15 months postoperatively, the patient continued to do well, with preserved alignment and fusion mass consolidation (Fig. 21.5a–c).

Salient Points/Pearls

- Goal of treatment: a stable limb that allows ambulation.
- Significant deformities require corrective fusions.

- Utilize more fixation than typical for nondiabetic/Charcot fusions.
- Be prepared to extend fusion to calcaneus.
- Progress slowly and recommend bracing with a CROW boot for at least 6 months as protection.

References

1. Blume PA, Sumpio B, Schmidt B, Donegan R. Charcot neuroarthropathy of the foot and ankle: diagnosis and management strategies. Clin Podiatr Med Surg. 2014;31(1):151–72.
2. Ramanujam CL, Stapleton JJ, Zgonis T. Diabetic charcot neuroarthropathy of the foot and ankle with osteomyelitis. Clin Podiatr Med Surg. 2014;31(4):487–92.
3. La Fontaine J, Lavery L, Jude E. Current concepts of Charcot foot in diabetic patients. Foot (Edinb). 2016;26:7–14.
4. Trepman E, Nihal A, Pinzur MS. Current topics review: Charcot neuroarthropathy of the foot and ankle. Foot Ankle Int. 2005;26(1):46–63.
5. Stapleton JJ, Zgonis T. Concomitant osteomyelitis and avascular necrosis of the talus treated with talectomy and tibiocalcaneal arthrodesis. Clin Podiatr Med Surg. 2013;30(2):251–6.

Chapter 22
Post-traumatic Ankle Arthropathy Treated with Arthrodesis

Matthew S. MacDougall, Daniel J. Gittings, and Jaimo Ahn

Clinical History

A 46-year-old man with a history of a traumatic ankle injury 30 years ago presented to the office with waxing and waning left ankle pain and discomfort. Over the previous year, his pain had substantially worsened. His symptoms include a grinding sensation and increased difficulty walking on a daily basis with pain affecting the medial, lateral, and anterior aspect of the ankle. He had no motor or sensory deficit. He was able to walk a few blocks despite the pain before needing

M.S. MacDougall, M.S.
Department of Biochemistry and Molecular Genetics, University of Illinois, Chicago, IL, USA

D.J. Gittings, M.D. • J. Ahn, M.D., Ph.D., F.A.C.S. (✉)
Department of Orthopaedic Surgery, University of Pennsylvania, Philadelphia, PA, USA
e-mail: jaimo.ahn@uphs.upenn.edu

N.C. Tejwani (ed.), *Fractures of the Foot and Ankle*,
DOI 10.1007/978-3-319-60456-5_22,

to stop with intermittent use of an ankle gauntlet-type brace and cane. Radiographs demonstrated post-traumatic degenerative changes of the left ankle joint.

Injury Films

Treatment Considerations

The patient had a history of ankle trauma as a teenager and ankle pain over the course of 30 years. His clinical history and radiographs were consistent with post-traumatic ankle arthritis in the setting of chronic ankle instability (Fig. 22.1). Given the long clinical course and increasing difficulty with walking, the primary goal was to restore a painless ankle. Given the patient's young age, activity level, and localized pain, he elected to undergo treatment with tibiotalar arthrodesis. Tibiotalar arthrodesis was the chosen treatment because of the procedure's ability to improve pain and to maintain

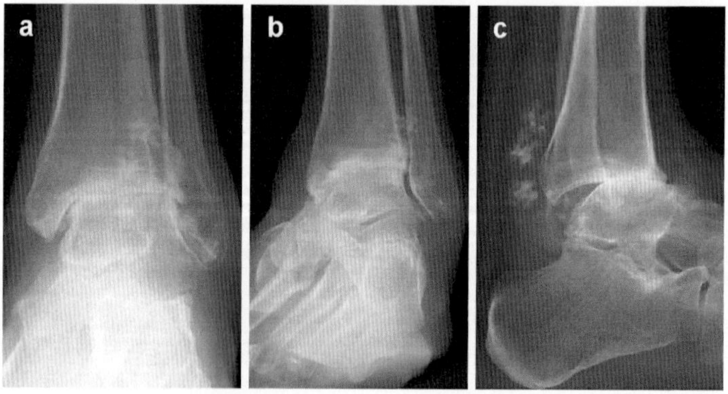

FIGURE 22.1 Preoperative (**a**) anterior-posterior, (**b**) mortise, and (**c**) lateral radiographs of the left ankle demonstrated post-traumatic degenerative changes including joint space narrowing and sclerosis along with anterior subluxation of the talus and, additionally, soft tissue calcification

durable functional motion through adjacent joints. Tibiotalar arthrodesis benefits from high success rates, and low rates of reoperation [1–12]. For this case, in order to allow extensile access to the joint (including calcifications), medial and lateral approaches with osteotomies of the fibula and medial malleolus were utilized.

Surgical Tact

Position: The patient was placed in a supine position with a bump under the left ipsilateral hip to internally rotate the ankle to assist in exposure of the lateral ankle.

Approach and osteotomy: First, an incision was made on the lateral aspect of the ankle superficial to the fibula curving anteriorly toward the fourth ray at the tip of the fibula. Sharp dissection was taken to the level of the fascia. The fascia overlying the fibula was incised and continued distally past the tip of the fibula providing access to the tibiotalar articulation, the proximal talus, and the sinus tarsi.

A distal fibula osteotomy was then performed, approximately 4 cm proximal to the distal tip of the fibula. The cut edge was beveled and some of the excised fibula was saved for later placement as local bone graft. Utilizing lateral and medial exposures, Kirschner wires were placed parallel to the joint in the AP view and perpendicular to the long axis of the tibia on the lateral view to guide the joint preparation. Osteotomy was utilized to remove the damaged cartilage and subchondral bone in linear planes on AP and lateral views for both the talus and distal tibia to allow for arthrodesis without shear planes despite some anterior bone loss.

The medial malleolus was then osteotomized and removed to allow for better joint access, to decrease increased prominence from shortening of the tibio-calcaneal distance, and to ensure relief of medial arthritic pain. The combination of bone cuts allowed neutral dorsiflexion, neutral coronal balance (Note: 5° of valgus is often stated to be acceptable or desirable), and slight external rotation.

Fixation: After verification of alignment and rotation using fluoroscopy, position was maintained by the placement of three guide wires (Fig. 22.2a). Two guide wires were placed through the talus, and into the distal tibia. The third guide wire was placed from the distal tibia into the talus. (Note: The sometimes recommended screw placement that we did not use for this case is directed proximal-posterior in the tibia to distal-anterior into the talar head.) Near cortices were predrilled and cannulated cancellous screws were placed. Placement of the first screw achieved compression across the arthrodesis site. The two additional screws provided additional compression, stability, and strength. Fluoroscopy was again used to confirm desired tibiotalar alignment and position of the hardware. The wounds were copiously irrigated with sterile saline and closed in a layered fashion over a drain.

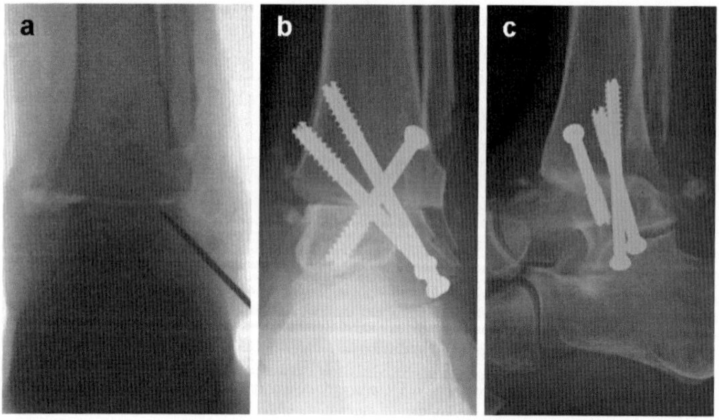

FIGURE 22.2 (**a**) Intraoperative fluoroscopic AP radiograph of the left ankle showing K-wire placement for cannulated screws. (**b** and **c**) AP and lateral radiographs of the left ankle immediately postoperatively demonstrating functional alignment and fixation of the tibiotalar joint

Postoperative Plan

Sterile dressings were applied and final plain radiographic images were taken (Fig. 22.2b, c). A splint was then applied for 2 weeks for soft tissue protection. The patient's activity status was recommended to be non-weight-bearing until wounds were healed and followed by touch-down weight-bearing until 6 weeks after surgery (with radiographic verification of maintained alignment) and finally full weight-bearing at 3 months. Protective CAM boot was utilized until pain free weight-bearing had been achieved just prior to 4 months after surgery.

Outcome

The patient's 16-month postoperative radiographs are shown in Fig. 22.3, which demonstrated consolidated tibiotalar fusion in functional alignment without hardware complication. Functionally, he completed a course of physical therapy during which he successfully advanced to full weight-bearing activity with no residual ankle pain and no visible limp with walking at up to moderate speeds.

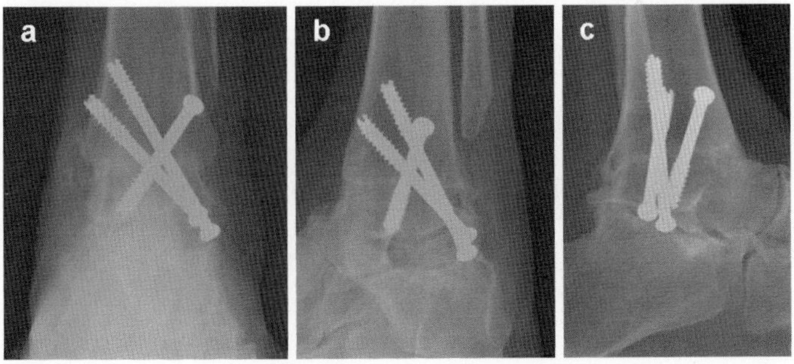

FIGURE 22.3 (**a–c**) 16-month postoperative AP, mortise, and lateral radiographs of the left ankle showing union of the tibiotalar joint

Salient Points/Pearls

- Trauma is the most common cause of ankle arthritis (70%) with the following types of injury being the most common: rotational fractures, recurrent ankle instability, and single ligamentous sprains with continued pain [13].
- Important determinants of surgical decision-making are the patient's pain, anatomy, and functional disability.
- Tibiotalar arthrodesis is indicated for post-traumatic ankle arthritis because of the procedure's ability to improve pain while maintaining functional motion through adjacent joints, durability for active/younger patients, high success rates, and low rates of reoperation [1–12].
- While tibiotalar arthrodesis is the gold standard for treatment of tibiotalar arthritis, total ankle replacement may be considered in patients with low functional demand and interest in attempted preservation of some tibiotalar motion [14].
- For successful tibiotalar arthrodesis to be achieved, the surgeon must consider the necessary soft tissue approach(es), bony access, strategy for joint preparation, fixation, and postoperative rehabilitation.
- The lateral, trans-fibular approach with an accessory medial trans-malleolar osteotomy is a highly versatile approach, but anterior, posterolateral, arthroscopic combined with percutaneous, and mini-open (smaller anteromedial and anterolateral) approaches may also be used [15].
- The optimal alignment of the ankle is neutral dorsiflexion, 0–5° of valgus, and rotation equal to or slightly externally rotated relative to the contralateral ankle [14].
- The type of internal fixation chosen may depend on ankle anatomy, deformity, and the amount of strength needed, but 3-screw fixation is associated with short time until union, low nonunion risk (5.6%), and minimal implant imprint [16].
- Plate or nail fixation is also reasonable as options to stabilize the arthrodesis until fusion is achieved and both provide greater construct strength than screws alone.

However, plates typically require greater soft tissue exposure and nails (with retrograde insertion) must also involve the subtalar joint; and both will typically leave a larger metallic surgical footprint.

- For long-term rehabilitation, patients must be advised of the likelihood of midfoot arthritis.

References

1. Ahlberg A, Henricson AS. Late results of ankle fusion. Acta Orthop Scand. 1981;52:103–5.
2. Anderson JG, Coetzee JC, Hansen ST. Revision ankle fusion using internal compression arthrodesis with screw fixation. Foot Ankle Int. 1997;18:300–9.
3. Buchner M, Sabo D. Ankle fusion attributable to posttraumatic arthrosis: a long-term followup of 48 patients. Clin Orthop Relat Res. 2003:155–64.
4. Cobb TK, Gabrielsen TA, Campbell DC 2nd, Wallrichs SL, Ilstrup DM. Cigarette smoking and nonunion after ankle arthrodesis. Foot Ankle Int. 1994;15:64–7.
5. Fitzgibbons TC. Arthroscopic ankle debridement and fusion: indications, techniques, and results. Instr Course Lect. 1999;48:243–8.
6. Jackson A, Glasgow M. Tarsal hypermobility after ankle fusion--fact or fiction? J Bone Joint Surg Br. 1979;61-b:470–3.
7. Kats J, van Kampen A, de Waal-Malefijt MC. Improvement in technique for arthroscopic ankle fusion: results in 15 patients. Knee Surg Sports Traumatol Arthrosc. 2003;11:46–9.
8. Kollig E, Esenwein SA, Muhr G, Kutscha-Lissberg F. Fusion of the septic ankle: experience with 15 cases using hybrid external fixation. J Trauma. 2003;55:685–91.
9. Marcus RE, Balourdas GM, Heiple KG. Ankle arthrodesis by chevron fusion with internal fixation and bone-grafting. J Bone Joint Surg Am. 1983;65:833–8.
10. Marsh JL, Rattay RE, Dulaney T. Results of ankle arthrodesis for treatment of supramalleolar nonunion and ankle arthrosis. Foot Ankle Int. 1997;18:138–43.
11. Moran CG, Pinder IM, Smith SR. Ankle arthrodesis in rheumatoid arthritis. 30 cases followed for 5 years. Acta Orthop Scand. 1991;62:538–43.

12. Said E, Hunka L, Siller TN. Where ankle fusion stands today. J Bone Joint Surg Br. 1978;60-b:211–4.
13. Saltzman CL, Salamon ML, Blanchard GM, Huff T, Hayes A, Buckwalter JA, Amendola A. Epidemiology of ankle arthritis: report of a consecutive series of 639 patients from a tertiary orthopaedic center. Iowa Orthop J. 2005;25:44–6.
14. Weatherall JM, Mroczek K, McLaurin T, Ding B, Tejwani N. Post-traumatic ankle arthritis. Bull Hosp Jt Dis. 2013;71:104–12.
15. Nihal A, Gellman RE, Embil JM, Trepman E. Ankle arthrodesis. Foot Ankle Surg. 2008;14:1–10.
16. Goetzmann T, Mole D, Jullion S, Roche O, Sirveaux F, Jacquot A. Influence of fixation with two vs. three screws on union of arthroscopic tibio-talar arthrodesis: comparative radiographic study of 111 cases. Orthop Traumatol Surg Res. 2016;102:651–6.

Index

N.C. Tejwani (ed.), *Fractures of the Foot and Ankle*,
DOI 10.1007/978-3-319-60456-5

Printed by Printforce, the Netherlands